DEPARTMENT OF AGRICULTURE AND FISHERIES FOR SCOTLAND

ADVISORY BULLETIN No. 9

The Shepherd's Guide

A Guide to the Diseases of Sheep and to
the Care and Training of Sheepdogs

Originally compiled by the late J. Russell Greig, CBE, PhD, MRCVS, FRSE.
Extensively revised by J. A. Watt, BSc, PhD, MRCVS,
Veterinary Investigation Officer in Charge, the Edinburgh School of Agriculture.
The Section on Training and Handling Sheepdogs
contributed by A. McDiarmid.

EDINBURGH   HER MAJESTY'S STATIONERY OFFICE   1971

R.BLEAY

SBN 11 490514 2

Contents

	Page
Preface	1
Disinfection and Antisepsis	
Lambing	3
Disinfection of Lambing Pens	3
The Care of Hypodermic Syringes	3
Vaccine and Serum Therapy	
Vaccines	5
Antiserum	5
Methods of Injection	
Dosing Gun Injuries	7
Combined Vaccines	7
Intraperitoneal Injection	8
Disease Problems in the Housing of Sheep	
Hoggs	
Pneumonia	9
Orf	9
Worms	9
Fluke	10
Lice	10
Ewes	10
Lambs	11
Abortion (Kebbing)	
Enzootic Abortion of Ewes (E. A. E., Kebbing)	12
Vibriosis	13
Toxoplasmosis	14
Tick-Borne Fever	14
Salmonellosis and Other Infections	15
Rotten Lambs	15
Border Disease	15
Listeriosis	15
Q Fever	16

Bacterial Infections

Lamb Dysentery	17
Enterotoxaemia (Pulpy Kidney Disease)	18
Black Disease	19
Big Head	20
Blackquarter	21
Braxy	22
Tetanus (Lockjaw)	23
Metritis (Inflammation)	24
Colibacillosis (Watery Mouth)	25
Liver Necrosis	26
Tick Pyaemia (Cripples)	27
Spinal Abscess (Paralysis)	28
Joint-Ill	28
Erysipelas Infection:	
Crippling or Arthritis (Stiff Lamb Disease)	29
Foot-Rot	30
Foot Abscess	33
Scad (Scald)	33
Johne's Disease (Paratuberculosis)	34
Actinobacillosis (Cruels; Grothel's)	36
Listeriosis (Circling Disease)	37
Acute or Gangrenous Mastitis (Udderclap)	38
Chronic Mastitis	39
Pneumonia	40
Mycotic Dermatitis	42
Strawberry Foot Rot	42
Fleece Rot (Canary Wool; Green Wool)	43
Innoculation Sepsis (Vaccination Blackquarter)	43

Virus and Rickettsial Diseases

Foot-and-Mouth Disease	45
Louping-Ill	46
Scrapie	48
Contagious Pustular Dermatitis (Orf)	50
Ulcerative Dermatosis	52
Periorbital Eczema (Eye Scab)	52
Sheep Pulmonary Adenomatosis (Jaagsiekte)	53
Tick-Borne Fever	54
Contagious Ophthalmia (Heather Blindness)	55
Entropion	56

Functional Disorders

Pine	57
Swayback	59
White Muscle Disease (Stiff Lamb Disease)	60
Double Scalp	61

Functional Disorders—continued

    Other Bone Conditions
        Rickets (Bent-leg) 62
        Dental Mal-Occlusion (Open Mouth) 63
        Osteomalacia (Cruban) 63
    Pregnancy Toxaemia (Twin Lamb Disease) 64
    Lambing Sickness (Milk Fever) 65
    Magnesium Deficiency:
        Hypomagnesaemia (Tetany) 67
    Yellowses 68
    Face Scab 69

Poisoning in Sheep
    Copper 70
    Kale and Rape 71
    Rhododendron 72

Miscellaneous Conditions
    Daft Lambs (Dafties) (Inherited Cortical Cerebellar Atrophy) . . 73
    Red Foot 73
    Border Disease 74
    Nasal Catarrh 75
    Prolapse of the Vagina 75
    Prolapse of the Intestines 75
    Cerebrocortical Necrosis (CCN) 75
    Urinary Calculi (Stone; Gravel) 76
    Bright Blindness 77
    Acidosis 77

Ecto-Parasites
    Ked Infestation 79
    Louse Infestation 79
    Sheep Scab 80
    Tick Infestation 82
    Cutaneous Myiasis (Blow-Fly Strike) 84
    Nose Maggot Infestation 87
    Dipping 88

Worm-Parasites
    Roundworms of the Alimentary Tract
        Parasitic Gastro-Enteritis 94
    Specific Infestations
        Nematodirus Disease (Nematodiriasis) . . . 97
        '*July Disease*' 98
        Haemonchus Contortus 98
        Chabertia Ovina 99

Worm–Parasites—continued

   Roundworms of the Respiratory Tract
      Parasitic or Verminous Pneumonia (Husk: Hoose). . . . 100
   Flat Worms (Trematodes or Flukes)
      Liver Fluke Infestation (Fascioliasis or Liver Rot) . . . 101
      Acute Type of Liver Fluke Infestation 103
      Chronic Type of Liver Fluke Infestation 104
   Flat Worms (Cestodes or Tapeworms)
      Tapeworm Infestation 106
      Coenurosis Cerebralis (*Sturdy; Gid; Turning Sickness*) . . . 107
      Hydatid Disease 108
      Bladder Worm 108
      Sheep 'Measles' 108
      Control of Tapeworm Cysts 109
      Coccidiosis 109

The Sheepdog
   Health and Welfare
      Feeding 111
      Housing 111
      Disease 112
      Parasites 112
      External Parasites 113

Training and Handling Sheepdogs
   Choosing a Dog 114
   Initial Training 114
   Obedience 115
   Introduction to Sheep 116
   Training with Sheep 117
   Gathering 118
   Driving 118
   Shedding 119
   Conclusion 119

Preface

One hundred and sixty years ago James Hogg published a book entitled 'The Shepherd's Guide on the Diseases of the Sheep'. The late Dr J. Russell Greig chose the same title for this handbook when the first edition was published in 1951. In his preface he stated that the book was primarily intended for the guidance of the shepherd. This principle has been carefully observed in the preparation of this edition and technical jargon has been reduced to a minimum. The aim throughout has been to provide information to give an understanding of the disease processes involved, with particular emphasis on methods of control. The book is not intended to act as a guide to 'do-it-yourself' diagnosis, however, and it must be emphasised that this diagnosis must be made by the veterinary surgeon. Only then is the information of real value.

While as much as possible of Dr Greig's original material and characteristic style has been left unchanged, it has been necessary—such is the advance of knowledge—to rewrite, in part at least, the majority of the items in the book and to include many conditions omitted in previous editions. The format has been slightly altered, it being thought advisable, for example, to place all types of abortion together rather than separate them according to the causal agent.

While it is believed that most of the conditions which have been identified in Scotland have been included, and reference made to others which have been recorded in other parts of Britain, the contents are not claimed to be a comprehensive review of every disease affecting sheep. It is, however, hoped that all conditions of importance in this country have been covered.

My thanks are due to those members of the Veterinary Investigation Services in Scotland who have helped with suggestions for alterations and additions and in particular to those who have edited and contributed individual items. Similarly, the invaluable help, contributions and advice from members of the staff of the Animal Diseases Research Association, Moredun Institute are gratefully acknowledged. My thanks are also due to Miss Anne Rodger for ready and valuable secretarial assistance.

I am particularly grateful to Dr J. T. Stamp for reading every item after revision, and for his continuing encouragement, advice and help.

J. A. WATT

Disinfection and Antisepsis

Until 1865, when Joseph Lister put into practice his germ theory of suppuration, the death-rate following surgical operation and even normal childbirth was appalling.

It had earlier been recognised that germs or microbes were all around and about us; on the ground we tread, the clothes we wear, the food we eat and the very air we breathe. Many of these microbes are harmless, some even beneficial, but others are dangerous to our well-being in that, given favourable opportunity, they can cause disease.

Lister showed that wound-sepsis (suppuration; putrefaction) was caused by the invasion of the injured tissues by germs and he also showed that these germs could be controlled by certain chemical agents of which carbolic acid was among the first to be applied; such substances are called 'antiseptics'. It was also proved that articles deliberately brought into contact with wounds, such as surgical instruments and wound dressings, could be 'sterilised' or 'disinfected' and so rendered safe by placing them in solutions of certain chemical agents or by immersing them in boiling water. This is because the germs of suppuration are destroyed, not only by certain chemicals but also, and relatively easily, by heat. So in brief, the 'Antiseptic Principle' is the prevention of suppurative microbes from entering a wound and the destruction or control of such microbes that have succeeded in entering the wound.

Although many shepherds clearly understand the principles of antisepsis and disinfection, these principles are often not applied, and much preventable loss of sheep life results from this failure. On the other hand, much injury results from the application of antiseptics that are in too strong concentration. The cresols and coal-tar acids are, among others, suitable disinfectants commonly used by shepherds. Many of these preparations, while useful when applied in proper concentration, are caustic and harmful to wounded tissues if applied too strong. There still exists a widespread, erroneous idea that the stronger the antiseptic solution the better, in that it will the more likely effect the destruction of microbes in the wound. This idea overlooks that fact that the process of rapid and satisfactory healing first requires that the wounded tissues are themselves healthy; many antiseptic applications although readily destructive to microbes are also injurious to the delicate tissue cells, and so seriously retard healing.

It is important, therefore, to use antiseptics which do not injure tissues even when used neat and there are many such preparations on the market. These differ markedly in smell and appearance from the traditional types but are effective and harmless.

The same principles apply to all preparations applied to skin wounds, maggot wounds and to the feet. Some preparations for foot-rot and scad are very caustic and painful and should never be used. Even recognised dressings such as formalin must be used at the recommended dilutions. In many cases dressing of wounds etc is best done, not by the application of disinfectants and antiseptics, but by the use of antibiotics such as penicillin which prevent bacteria multiplying without in any way retarding the healing process.

LAMBING

Disinfection and cleanliness are extremely important when assisting a ewe to lamb. To avoid infection in the flock, washing of the hands and forearms should be scrupulously carried out before and after lambing or handling any infective material. Soap also makes a useful lubricant for the arm although the use of barrier and mild antiseptic creams is recommended. Pessaries which are placed in the womb after an assisted lambing are useful where any damage has been done and powerful antibiotics in this form can be obtained. Your veterinary surgeon will advise on this point. Such medication is always indicated when dead or, more important, 'rotten' lambs are delivered.

DISINFECTION OF LAMBING PENS

Though lambing ewes, unlike other farm animals, are not usually housed, this practice is now growing. Where this is done it is important to empty the house of sheep and disinfect the pens after each lambing. The method to be adopted, however, varies with the system, so recommendations which would fit all conditions cannot be laid down.

However, on most farms, lambing still takes place in pens and attention must be paid to these if infections of the newborn lamb are to be avoided. Such pens usually consist of temporary erections of wooden rails, straw, etc, and as these cannot be readily disinfected it is best to use a different site each year, the straw being burned and the rails creosoted. Permanent lambing pens should be constructed with smooth walls and floor for ease of cleaning and disinfection, which is best done initially with strong hot washing soda followed by an approved disinfectant.

Infection can, however, build up during an ordinary lambing season, resulting in outbreaks of joint-ill and coliform infections in the second-half of lambing. The trouble can be avoided by having sufficient pens and a large enough enclosure so that only half is required for the early part of the lambing, the clean part being used later in the season, or whenever disease appears. Permanent pens should be cleaned as already described though this is difficult during lambing. The only alternative if disease appears is to move the remaining ewes to temporary quarters.

THE CARE OF HYPODERMIC SYRINGES

After use the interior of the barrel of the syringe and the needles should be cleansed by alternatively drawing up and ejecting clean, cold water several times.

The syringe and needles should then be sterilised by boiling for ten minutes. The instrument should be taken to pieces for sterilisation; if boiled as a complete unit unequal expansion of the glass is apt to occur, with consequent risk of breakage.

After their sterilisation the syringe and needles are wrapped up in a dry cloth that has been sterilised by boiling, or replaced in the metal container-case, provided that this also has been sterilised by boiling.

The several types of multiple syringe available require special care because of the valves, etc. The maker's instructions for cleansing and sterilising should be carefully carried out immediately after use. Never leave any syringe uncleaned and unsterilised overnight even though it is to be used next day.

Vaccine and Serum Therapy

A number of infectious diseases of sheep can be controlled by immunising the animals with a vaccine or an antiserum. There are important differences between the two which should be understood if they are to be used correctly and effectively.

VACCINES
When an animal is inoculated with an infective agent or its products (toxins), modified by heat or chemicals so as to be incapable of causing disease, the body does not distinguish this from a natural attack of the disease and produces 'immune bodies' or 'antibodies' which will neutralise the germ or its toxin. The body, however, requires time to do this and in many cases two injections separated by an interval are necessary before the animal is well protected, *eg* in the use of 'combined vaccines', so vaccines are used to prevent disease which is expected in the future and they must be administered sufficiently long before the period of risk for the animal to develop a high level of immunity. Such an immunity resulting from vaccination lasts for a long time and is readily boosted by a single further injection of vaccine, *eg* in the injection of the ewe annually with pulpy kidney/lamb dysentery vaccine.

ANTISERUM
When an animal is vaccinated repeatedly the blood serum becomes very rich indeed in the antibodies against the disease organisms from which the vaccine was made. If such serum is withdrawn from this animal and is then injected into a susceptible animal it will carry these antibodies with it and will immediately make the receiving animal immune. The same 'donor' mechanism works when a lamb takes the ewe's colostrum (first milk), which is very rich in any antibodies the ewe has, either as a result of natural infection or of vaccination. It is very important that the lamb gets this milk in the first twelve hours of life, as after this its ability to absorb antibodies rapidly declines. This immunity, however, though immediate, lasts only till the antibodies are lost or used, usually in a few weeks, and if the animal has not been exposed to the natural disease in this time it is as susceptible as ever. Serum, therefore, is employed only when disease has broken out unexpectedly and the vaccine would take too long to work, as in pulpy kidney disease and black disease. Serum can of course be used to prevent disease where the period of risk is short as in lamb dysentery, but more usually it is used in 'fire brigade' action.

Methods of Injection

All inoculations mean that foreign material is deliberately introduced past the body's first line of defence—the skin. It is very important then that only the inoculum is injected and that no damage is done to the tissues under the skin which would allow any stray germs to get a hold and cause suppuration and even death. Every year there are outbreaks of this type—sometimes with heavy losses—which could have been avoided with proper common-sense precautions. Another factor is that many modern vaccines contain substances called 'adjuvants' which heighten the effect of the vaccine and are, in fact, necessary to stimulate the desired immunity. These adjuvants tend to remain at the site of inoculation for some time in the form of areas of discolouration in the flesh, or even small sterile abscesses. Most shepherds will have noticed such abscesses at clipping when they are readily damaged. In sheep destined eventually for slaughter such blemishes can be important, often necessitating unsightly trimming which reduces the value of the carcase. This loss can be greatly reduced by giving the inoculation in a carefully selected site.

Vaccines are supplied as 'sterile', meaning that they do not contain germs which are capable of causing suppuration and inflammation. Nearly all outbreaks of infection can be traced to contamination of the syringe or the bottle in use. First then, choose a dry day for all inoculations, with dry clean sheep and dry pens. The next important point is the location for the job: for ease of handling and reduction of stress on both sheep and man this is best done in the standing position either in a crush or, where labour permits, by having an adequate number of catchers. The person carrying out the injections should handle the sheep as little as possible. The inoculator should lean over the sheep, pick up a fold of skin by the wool and gently insert the needle almost parallel to the side of the sheep—needle pointing downwards—so that the point of the needle comes to rest just below the skin two ins above and behind the elbow. A slight variation in the site is not of great importance provided this area is used. All sheep should be vaccinated on the same side. If proper precautions to exclude dirt and germs are taken, the site for serum injections is not important. For example, the shepherd catching and injecting lambs against lamb dysentery will usually inject in the inside of the thigh.

Where the single dose syringe is being used a sterile needle should be pushed into the vaccine bottle and left there. Never use the same needle for withdrawing vaccine from the bottle and injecting the sheep. Should such a needle penetrate a tiny abscess the germs will be washed into the vaccine bottle and will infect every sheep injected from that bottle. Use a freshly boiled needle for every bottle, change to a freshly boiled syringe for every bottle and use a sterile needle for every score or so of sheep. Syringes can be rinsed in clean water, dismantled and boiled up over a primus stove for use again immediately. For the odd injection occasionally needed, plastic disposable syringes are useful. These are used once then discarded. They are supplied sterilised in a sealed pack.

With multiple syringes the main points are to flush with boiled cold water after each bottle and to clean and sterilise according to instructions after each period of use. If these methods are followed there is little risk of 'inoculation blackquarter' (*see* page 43) and carcasses are easily trimmed if this is necessary because of vaccine blemishes.

DOSING GUN INJURIES

Though not so frequent as they were in the days when boluses or tablets were commonly used, deaths still result from damage to the throat through careless or over-enthusiastic use of the dosing gun. Injured sheep appear normal for a few days after the dosing, then are seen to be very sick and die from five to ten days later. Guns should be free from rough edges and should not be pushed too far back. Never dose a struggling sheep and take plenty of time. There is little point in setting up records for numbers dosed if some reject the medicine and others die from throat injuries.

COMBINED VACCINES

The vaccines developed for use against specific diseases will be mentioned under each disease. There is, however, one group of vaccines which merits special treatment and that is the group which protects against the 'anaerobic' diseases. Sheep are peculiarly susceptible to diseases caused by this group of organisms, so named because they can be grown in the laboratory only in the absence of oxygen. The best known are pulpy kidney, braxy, lamb dysentery and black disease, but others of the group are blackquarter, tetanus (lockjaw) and 'struck'. Formerly an exact diagnosis of the type of microbe causing the disease was essential, for each and every one had its own vaccine. Now, however, methods have been developed of combining these vaccines without loss of efficiency and vaccines are available containing two, three, four and even seven components.

Whichever vaccine is chosen as the most suitable for the particular flock, the basic principles are the same in that two injections are required at an interval of not less than one month, with booster doses once annually. The advantages of building up a fully protected flock must be considered and here again the basic principles are the same. The programme should commence when the numbers on the farm are at their minimum, *ie* in the autumn. Every animal is given two injections at an interval of at least one month and the in-lamb ewes are given a booster dose some 14 days before lambing is due to begin. This dose gives a high level of protective antibodies in the colostrum or first milk which, it is claimed, will protect the lambs for from eight to ten weeks against lamb dysentery and pulpy kidney disease. The lambs are given their first injection at six to eight weeks and those which are being retained are given a second injection after at least four weeks. The spring booster dose is usually all that is required thereafter, though where black disease is prevalent a booster dose may be necessary in the autumn. This procedure avoids the labour of giving each lamb serum at birth, as well as protecting the ewes. This is the outline of one scheme but the method can be varied. Suppliers of vaccine provide recommendations for the use of their product and the choice of product and method is a matter for discussion with your veterinary surgeon.

INTRAPERITONEAL INJECTION

More recently a development of the multiple vaccine has resulted in a product which it is claimed will protect sheep from clostridial disease for a period of years. This vaccine is 'intraperitoneal', *ie* given by direct injection into the abdomen, and should therefore be administered by a veterinary surgeon. The vaccine should not be used in pregnant animals. Though the overall protection is of long duration, a special vaccine is given under the skin to the pregnant protected ewe to boost the protective level of her colostrum; this vaccine is given to the animals between twelve and two weeks before lambing. This procedure is claimed to protect the lambs—provided they get an adequate feed of colostrum in the first few hours of life—for at least 16 weeks. The vaccine can be used in sheep over 10 weeks of age. Rams are given a booster dose every two years.

The following advantages are claimed for intraperitoneal vaccine. Only a single injection is needed to protect sheep and sensitise them to subsequent doses of the subcutaneous booster vaccine. A single dose of 2 ml protects for several years and the pre-lambing booster dose of vaccine can be given well in advance of lambing, thus the handling of ewes heavy in lamb is avoided. Much greater antibody concentrations are stimulated by the intraperitoneal vaccine than by the traditional adjuvant vaccines and fewer injections are required. This results in a saving of time and effort and an overall reduction in labour costs, while the use of the non-adjuvant vaccine for booster effect reduces the risk of carcase blemish. The latitude permissible in the timing of injections gives this system sufficient flexibility for adaptation to all types of sheep husbandry.

Disease Problems in the Housing of Sheep

The practice of housing sheep, particularly hoggs, is not new but until recently it has been out of use for so many years that the know-how has been lost. Reviving interest in the practice, however, justifies some comment on the factors which may affect health. These differ considerably between hoggs and in-lamb ewes.

HOGGS

The only hazards of an infectious or parasitic nature which have to be guarded against in the hoggs are pneumonia, orf, worms, fluke and lice.

Pneumonia

As can be seen from the section on pneumonia (*see* page 40) we still have much to learn about this disease, but there is little doubt that in the context of housing, ventilation is the major factor. Outbreaks of apparently infectious pneumonia can occur even when the ventilation seems ideal, but this is not surprising when it is considered that similar outbreaks can occur out-of-doors, although comparatively rarely. But faulty ventilation can cause a great deal of trouble and loss, so it is very important to obtain expert advice in constructing and adapting buildings. The general principle to be aimed at is to have plenty of air circulating above, with no particularly draughty or sheltered corners at sheep level. As each case requires individual consideration it is not possible to be more exact. Do not attempt to erect a new building or adapt an older one without making use of the specialist advisory services in this field.

Orf

Where this disease occurs, or has occurred naturally, the animals should be vaccinated shortly before housing, if this has not already been done. If, however, orf is unknown on the farm, vaccination is not advisable as the vaccine is live and its use might actually introduce infection.

Worms

The hoggs will undoubtedly be carrying a burden of worms and as they will not be exposed to infection inside they should be dosed when they are brought in, or within three weeks. A full dose of an effective non-toxic remedy should be given. If an outside run is provided, however, housed hoggs can be heavily infected and must be dosed regularly.

Fluke

This infestation will only be important in flukey areas, but in such areas the ordinary routine dosing should be supplemented by a dose six to eight weeks after housing. The drug used in this dosing should be free from danger in concentrate-fed animals and your vet should be consulted about the drug which may be most safely used.

Lice

These parasites can be a considerable problem in hoggs, both housed and on free range. To obtain the maximum freedom, the hoggs should be carefully dipped as close to the housing date as possible and allowed to dry before being brought in. It is important that this dipping be carried out with great care.

Hoggs can be run in numbers up to 100 or even more in the pen but the pen must have no protruding posts—if these are present, shoulder boards should be fitted. The floor should be dry and firm. Water should be supplied so that it keeps fresh and cool. Automatic drinking bowls are not really suitable as hill sheep rarely use them. It may be necessary to arrange to have the water actually flowing in some cases. It is essential to have sufficient trough space so that all the hoggs can feed simultaneously, otherwise the shyer animals will suffer from malnutrition.

Hoggs straight from the hill are easily startled and care must be taken for a few days otherwise crushing may occur. Once they are used to their attendant there will be little trouble but strangers and dogs may still cause alarm.

EWES

The remarks previously made about ventilation apply equally to the houses for the ewes. Ewes should be wormed when brought in and on fluke areas should be dosed for this parasite four to six weeks after housing as well as at the time of housing.

The numbers which it is advisable to have per pen are, however, very different, as no more than 10–20 ewes should share the same pen in order to control the spread of contagious disease which is much more important in the ewe than in the hogg. Even orf can result in losses amongst the ewes from mastitis, while if one of the infectious forms of abortion appeared and there were no barrier to its spread amongst large groups of ewes, a major catastrophe could result.

The ewes should be selected for their pens partly on age and condition and partly on their expected lambing date, if they are to be lambed indoors. Gimmers, for example, should be housed together, apart from the ewes, to avoid bullying and to make sure they get their ration. Thin ewes, if penned in one group, can be fed more generously. The idea of grouping by the expected lambing date is to avoid long-drawn-out lambing in any one pen as this not infrequently results in the build-up of infection for the newly born lamb, *eg* coliform infections, joint-ill and navel-ill.

It is better to lamb the ewe in the pen she has occupied rather than to remove her to a lambing pen, as this puts a stress on the ewe with, on occasion, unfortunate side effects.

There are, of course, other points which require consideration—vaccinations for example—so it is advisable for any farmer thinking of adopting housing to consult his veterinary surgeon and the College farm buildings adviser for his area before beginning his planning. If housing ewes becomes more common, we will undoubtedly find other conditions which require attention, but there is sufficient knowledge available to reduce the risks and make the practice feasible from a health view-point.

LAMBS

Lambs present the usual problems though the risks involved in infective disease are, of course, favoured by the intensification. For this reason foresight in penning the ewes is essential. Lambs retained inside for fattening do not run any risk from worm infestation but coccidiosis can be a problem. This disease is not very responsive to treatment once symptoms have developed, so efforts should be directed to control by prophylactic measures on which your veterinary surgeon will advise.

Abortion (Kebbing)

The term 'kebbing' implies the birth of dead lambs either at term or prematurely, or of live, premature, weak lambs. While it would not be true to say that the cause of outbreaks of kebbing can be identified in all cases, the picture is now much clearer than formerly, with the identification of certain infective agents and the development of tests to confirm their presence.

ENZOOTIC ABORTION OF EWES (E.A.E., KEBBING)

This condition is one of the most important causes of loss in south-east Scotland but, contrary to former belief, the disease is by no means confined to this area, having been recorded in practically every county in England and in many overseas countries. The disease is essentially confined to lowground flocks and has not been found in a true hill flock. This is certainly because of the difference in management at lambing and cannot be attributed to any resistance in the hill breeds.

CAUSE Enzootic abortion results from infection with a large virus which can be seen with the ordinary microscope. The foetal membrane or afterbirth is the tissue affected and here the virus produces changes which are quite characteristic and usually readily recognised on naked eye examination.

The disease itself is characterised by the birth of dead and weakly lambs in the last 14 days of pregnancy. Abortions may occasionally occur as long as three to four weeks before the ewe is due to lamb, but these are exceptional. The dead lambs are almost invariably well developed and fresh and apparently normal but the placenta or afterbirth—which is usually voided uneventfully—is thickened and discoloured. In a very few cases where the afterbirth is retained the ewe may develop inflammation of the womb, but this is rare. Ewes recover well and, in fact, usually milk well enough to rear a lamb. These ewes are then immune and will conceive and lamb naturally after the next mating.

Infection is believed to spread chiefly at lambing time, the products of birth and discharges from affected ewes being the main source. It is obvious, therefore, that the ewe should be isolated at once and the foetus and placenta burned. It is quite wrong to put her out with the hoggs as she may infect them and they will then abort at their first pregnancy. For the same reason it is inadvisable to twin on a ewe lamb which may be kept for breeding, as there is some evidence that even at this early age the infection can be picked up, to remain latent, till in due course she becomes pregnant.

On the other hand the practice sometimes adopted of selling aborted ewes is not advisable as the infection will never be eliminated this way. Many infected ewes will not keb but will give birth to live lambs and so will not be noticed.

They can, however, infect other ewes. As such ewes can be depended on to lamb normally next season they should be retained. There is no evidence that the rams are involved in any way.

As is to be expected with this method of spread, the second crop is usually the worst affected though, on occasion, the gimmers are the chief sufferers. The overall incidence in a flock varies considerably, being high (20–30 per cent) when first introduced, then settling down at 4–5 per cent.

DIAGNOSIS This is based on the history of the flock and confirmed in the laboratory by demonstrating the causal virus from the placenta. It is very important that this placenta be included when a lamb is sent to the laboratory. A blood test taken up to several weeks after the abortion will also confirm the disease, but samples from several affected ewes should be submitted. This blood test will not detect ewes which are harbouring the infection but have not yet aborted, so it cannot be used to eliminate infection from the flock.

CONTROL This is by attention to management as suggested above, but vaccination is essential. The vaccine is given to the gimmers two to three weeks before mating and one injection is believed to protect for life. As the disease is essentially one of fairly intensive husbandry the importance of anticipating its occurrence and taking steps to control it are particularly important when ewes are housed. Unfortunately, the other conditions which cause abortion are not influenced by the vaccine against this disease and the vaccine is often condemned as a failure when abortions occur in vaccinated flocks. These outbreaks frequently have other causes and it is important to realise that every outbreak is not attributable to this particular virus.

VIBRIOSIS

Again the only symptom is abortion or kebbing. Unlike enzootic abortion, however, the disease does not tend to persist in a flock, an abortion 'storm' being succeeded in the following year by an uneventful lambing, or at most one or two abortions. The disease is known wherever sheep are kept.

CAUSE The causal microbe is known as *Vibrio foetus* and a related microbe is responsible for infertility and abortion in cattle. Abortions take place in the last six weeks of pregnancy and tend to be earlier in pregnancy than those due to enzootic abortion. The disease in sheep, however, is not a cause of infertility nor is it venereally transmitted, infection being acquired by ingestion.

The aborted lamb is often less well developed than in enzootic abortion and decomposing and mummified lambs are not infrequently seen. The afterbirth, unlike enzootic abortion, shows few visible lesions.

The source of these infections is not clear but it is possible that carrier animals exist, though the ram does not appear to play any part in an outbreak. Incidents of this nature do not occur sufficiently often to justify the development of vaccine, but where very intensive husbandry is practised, with housing of ewes, the position may need to be reviewed. The incidence can be very high in some outbreaks—over 50 per cent—but, as has been said, the disease does not tend to recur. Where an outbreak has been confirmed early, the use of antibiotics has been claimed to help. These, however, must never be given except under veterinary advice.

DIAGNOSIS This is based on history, the appearance of the foetus and membranes and demonstration of the microbe in the laboratory from the afterbirth and stomach contents of the lamb. Blood tests are unsatisfactory in this disease.

TOXOPLASMOSIS

This disease has only recently been recognised as being of importance in sheep abortion. The cause is a protozoan parasite *Toxoplasma gondii*. Many sheep appear to be infected without showing any signs of infection. The means of spread is unknown but it would appear wise to treat the condition like any other infectious disease. The foetuses are often small and dried up with dry brownish membranes. The cotyledons or buttons often show characteristic white pinhead spots which have given the condition the name of 'white spot abortion'.

DIAGNOSIS This is not always easy but is based on the recovery of the toxoplasma after inoculating mice with extracts from the afterbirth or tissues from the aborted foetus. The infection takes four to six weeks before cysts can be recognised in the brains of the mice. A serological test is helpful but not diagnostic as many non-aborting sheep carry the infection. Microscopic examination of tissues from the lamb is also useful.

CONTROL As the method of spread and infection is unknown, it is not possible to suggest methods of controlling this condition.

TICK-BORNE FEVER

One of the more spectacular effects of this disease (*see* page 54) is abortion in unacclimatised sheep. Abortion can take place during the last six weeks of pregnancy and possibly is the result of the prolonged high temperature of the affected ewe. The disease shows up under fairly well-defined conditions. The first is when gimmers and ewes from tick-free pastures are introduced to an infected hill, so that they encounter the tick and its accompanying disease for the first time in late pregnancy. The second is where a hill has been recently lightly infested with ticks, with the result that many ewes have no immunity: and lastly on hills either lightly infested or only locally infested, with the result, particularly when hoggs have been wintered away, that a number of the young stock encounter the disease for the first time as pregnant gimmers.

DIAGNOSIS This is based on the history, a knowledge of the area and, on occasion, the demonstration of the causal organism in blood smears from aborted ewes. The mere fact that the ewe can be shown to be carrying the disease is not of value, as once a sheep has become infected the disease is present in the blood for a year or more.

CONTROL   This is based on trying to ensure that all young stock are exposed to tick bite before they become in-lamb. It is important to remember that one tick is enough to carry the disease. Ewes from tick-free areas should never be put on tick-infested pasture.

SALMONELLOSIS AND OTHER INFECTIONS

Organisms of the salmonella group which cause food poisoning in man and scour in calves can cause losses amongst lambing ewes. While there is a specific salmonella associated with sheep abortion, this appears to be confined to southern England. The chief importance of this type of abortion is that it is accompanied by a fairly high death-rate in the ewes from inflammation of the womb and resultant general infection. For this reason early abortions, particularly if ewes are sick, should be viewed with caution and veterinary advice sought at once. As these organisms can cause disease in man strict personal hygiene is of great importance.

CONTROL   The disease is uncommon and does not seem to persist in the flock. Treatment is a matter for the veterinary surgeon and is directed to saving the affected ewes and preventing the spread of infection.

ROTTEN LAMBS

No definite infection appears to be associated with this condition though the dead foetus is often invaded by organisms of the clostridial group. The lambs are usually well developed but have become infected with organisms of putrefaction after death in the womb. The causes of such deaths are usually obscure but it is believed that many result from a subclinical toxaemia (*see* pregnancy toxaemia). Care in management and feeding may therefore limit losses from this cause. The major importance of this condition is death of the ewe from 'inflammation' after lambing. Some ewes may be saved by very early treatment.

BORDER DISEASE

One of the effects of this disease is the birth of premature lambs. The disease itself has been recently suspected in Scotland and in view of its apparent infectious nature it must be considered in this context. The actual cause is not known.

LISTERIOSIS

Though infection with the organism *listeria monocytogenes* is usually manifested in adult sheep by 'circling disease' (*see* page 37), the microbe has been incriminated in abortion. Its importance lies in its ability to cause severe and even fatal disease in the human and, together with Q. fever (*see* below), presents an excellent reason for care in handling kebs or abortions and emphasises the need for careful personal hygiene at lambing.

The disease can only be diagnosed in the laboratory by isolation of the causal microbe.

Q. FEVER

While this peculiarly named disease has not definitely been proved to cause abortion, the causal microbe *Rickettsia burneti* has been frequently isolated from sheep abortions and afterbirths. The organism, which is readily diagnosed in the laboratory from the afterbirth, can cause an unpleasant and highly infectious lung disease in man.

Other outbreaks occur in which a diagnosis cannot be made and, though uncommon, they can cause heavy loss on occasion. One difficulty in investigating such outbreaks is that they do not occur twice on the same farm and in fact a year or two may pass between outbreaks. The variety of causes involved, however, underlines the need for early and accurate diagnosis where abortions occur.

Bacterial Infection

LAMB DYSENTERY

Lamb dysentery is a highly contagious disease affecting young lambs during the first or, less commonly, the second week of life. The disease is localised in its distribution but has been recognised for many years, particularly in the Border counties. During the early half of the century the condition apparently increased in virulence and in extent but in the last 20 years it has become increasingly rare, probably as a result of the widespread use of efficient vaccines and sera.

CAUSE The causal organism is a member of the Clostridial group of anaerobic germs which cause so many of the diseases of sheep and is known as *Clostridium welchii* (type B). The disease only occurs when the lamb swallows this specific organism.

CONDITIONS OF OCCURRENCE Often the disease exists on affected farms for two or three years with only a few lambs becoming affected, usually near the end of lambing, but later the incidence suddenly increases and, upon occasion, 50 per cent of the lambs may be lost if diagnosis and preventive inoculations are not carried out. In recently affected flocks, usually only a few lambs are affected in the early part of lambing, but as this continues more and more lambs are infected. This is probably due to the great increase in the numbers of germs in the soil and pens.

SYMPTOMS In less acute cases the lamb is dull, lags behind the ewe and refuses to suck. The abdominal wall is tense and painful on pressure and diarrhoea is present, often with blood in the motions. These are yellow at first but soon become chocolate coloured. The disease is almost invariably fatal in one to three days. Occasionally, lambs are found dead without symptoms having been noticed.

POST-MORTEM FINDINGS In very acute cases inflammation varies from slight to marked, involving the whole intestine. In the more typical, less acute type, there are necrotic ulcers in the bowel. Loops of the bowel may be dark red in colour and sticking together.

PREVENTION There is no cure but the disease can be prevented by two methods. The first is by vaccination of the ewe, and lamb dysentery vaccine is present in most combined vaccines (*see* page 7). A booster injection 14 days or so before lambing is essential every year, while gimmers are vaccinated in the autumn also. The lamb must obtain the first milk early in life for this to be effective.

SERUM INJECTION   Where vaccination of the ewes is not carried out lambs are given hyper-immune antiserum as soon after birth as possible but in any case within 24 hours. The short immunity is sufficient to carry the lamb over the danger period. The anti-lamb dysentery sera now produced usually protect against pulpy kidney disease also.

On hill farms, ewe vaccination is the usual method because of the difficulty of catching every lamb on the hill in time, but with the greatly increased use of combined vaccines fewer lowground farms now use the serum method.

It is of interest to note that when the disease was being investigated at the Moredun Institute of the Animal Diseases Research Association many years ago the scientists first ascribed the disease to *Escherichia coli*. The interest lies in the fact that this organism is a much more common cause of death in young lambs at present than is lamb dysentery and it is probable that many of the cases investigated were, in fact, coli infections.

ENTEROTOXAEMIA (Pulpy Kidney Disease)

As the first name suggests the cause of the disease is located in the bowel. When conditions are suitable, the microbe *Clostridium welchii* (type D)—a close relation of the microbe causing lamb dysentery—multiplies at an enormous rate and produces large quantities of a toxin or poison which, when absorbed into the bloodstream of the sheep, causes death in a very short time. Sheep of all ages are affected.

CONDITIONS OF OCCURRENCE   The conditions which lead to the rapid growth of this microbe occur when quantities of rich semi-digested food are passed into the true stomach and bowel, so it most commonly occurs in the best thriving animals, or animals which are beginning to thrive after dosing or a change of pasture. The disease occurs in sheep of all ages, including lambs a few days old, but is most common in the six-week to one-year-old animals.

As one would expect with a disease dependent on nutrition, it tends to occur seasonally, though deaths resulting from it can happen at any time of the year. The first peak is seen when the lambs are six weeks to three months of age, when the grass is at its best and subject to periods of rapid growth and when a spell of warm damp weather follows a cold dry spell. This can result in deaths in the ewes as well as the lambs, the latter getting a flush of milk as well as extra grass. Too sudden a change from poor to rich pasture can have exactly the same effect and it is well recognised that every effort should be made to make this kind of change gradual.

While deaths may occur sporadically throughout the summer the next 'peak' in incidence is usually experienced when the weaned lambs get over the check of weaning and are moved to clean pasture, *eg* stubble or rape. At this time of the year the disease is often confused with braxy, but the two are readily differentiated by a veterinary surgeon on post-mortem examination. Acidosis and acute pasteurella pneumonia can also cause confusion.

In flocks where vaccination is not carried out ewe lambs may be affected when box feeding is begun in winter and it is in this group that the losses may again become important.

SYMPTOMS   Animals are usually found dead or in convulsions.

POST-MORTEM FINDINGS   The name of the disease is derived from the appearance of the kidneys shortly after death. Usually, but not always, these organs are soft and pulpy with blood splashes on them. There is usually an excess of clear fluid in the heart sac and here also a 'chickenfat' clot is commonly found. Kidneys, however, quickly decompose in diseases other than pulpy kidney and fluid round the heart is common in tetany and black disease, so laboratory tests may be necessary to ensure that the right preventive measures are adopted.

DIAGNOSIS   This then is based on the history, the post-mortem findings and laboratory tests on newly-dead animals.

PREVENTION AND CONTROL   The disease can be prevented by the correct use of vaccines and antiserum. Disease in the young lamb is controlled by double vaccination of the ewe, with the second or booster dose shortly before lambing. This is claimed to protect the lamb for from eight to twelve weeks. The lamb can be protected for up to nine months and perhaps longer by vaccination, as is claimed for the intraperitoneal vaccine. In an emergency, serum will give immediate protection for two or three weeks. Management measures are also successful, such as docking and castrating the lambs or moving them to poor pasture, both of which methods give the necessary check. Even bringing the lambs in and handling them for vaccination may give sufficient check. There is no doubt, however, that intelligent use of vaccine is the most reliable method.

Other diseases can be caused by the same conditions which result in deaths from pulpy kidney disease, *eg* acute pasteurellosis and acidosis, so vaccination does not provide an umbrella under which bad management can be practised with impunity.

BLACK DISEASE

This is another of the group of diseases caused by microbes of the Clostridial group. This microbe is called *Clostridium oedematiens* (type B) and in true black disease it affects the liver of the sheep. In this particular condition spores which have been picked up by the grazing sheep come to rest in the liver, where they are harmless until the liver is damaged by numbers of tiny flukes boring into the liver substance. As this happens in autumn and early winter the disease is very seasonal, occurring usually from September to February.

CONDITIONS OF OCCURRENCE   True black disease occurs where fluke is a parasite. Numbers of fluke are, of course, dependent on the numbers of the tiny mud snail which acts as the intermediate host, so the disease is usually worst after wet summers which favour the development of large numbers of snails. However, sheep may die from sheer numbers of fluke and this is difficult to differentiate from black disease. Severe frost tends to reduce the incidence. The organism can, however, cause death in the absence of fluke from either a form of black disease or a blackquarter-like condition.

SYMPTOMS The disease kills very rapidly once the microbe begins to grow and animals are seldom, if ever, seen ill. The affected sheep is commonly found on its brisket as if asleep without any sign of convulsions or struggling, though it might have appeared in perfect health two or three hours earlier.

POST-MORTEM FINDINGS Signs of the disease are readily seen in an animal examined within two to three hours of death, but later they are destroyed by putrefaction. The liver is very dark with soft mushy patches or with greyish areas of varying size surrounded by a dark ring. Fluid, which is often blood-stained, is found in the heart sac. The diagnosis is not always easy, however, particularly when it has to be differentiated from death following massive invasion of fluke. It can be readily confirmed in the fresh carcase by laboratory tests.

DIAGNOSIS This is dependent on skilled post-mortem differentiation from braxy and pulpy kidney disease with which it is often confused. Braxy is, however, rare in the usual age group affected—two years and older.

PREVENTION AND CONTROL When the disease is diagnosed and deaths are occurring, serum must be used. This should be combined with an injection of vaccine which is repeated in a month's time. When combined vaccines are used properly the animals will be immune, as most such vaccines include immunity against this disease. As a single dose of vaccine is commonly given to gimmers in the autumn with no further injection till lambing, it is important that where black disease occurs a first injection should be given in late July or early August so that the autumn injection will protect the animal over the danger period. A booster dose to the ewes may be advisable in bad years and the association of such years with weather conditions has enabled the Ministry of Agriculture to issue a forecast of the likely incidence of fluke. This can be useful in indicating when such a booster dose should be considered.

While full use should be made of the vaccine, management measures must not be neglected. Every possible step should be taken to control the snail host and these measures are described in the section dealing with fluke.

BIG HEAD

While this disease is not very common in this country it does occur amongst young rams, usually in isolated cases but occasionally several animals may be affected.

CAUSE The disease is due to local infection by the same germ which causes black disease—*Clostridium oedematiens*. The condition tends to be more common in areas where black disease occurs, probably because of the prevalence of the organism.

CONDITIONS OF OCCURRENCE The fact that most cases are seen in rams is probably the result of fighting. *Clostridium oedematiens* grows readily in damaged tissue and can gain access either through small wounds or from spores already in the tissues.

SYMPTOMS   The first symptom is a fairly rapid swelling of the whole head as a result of the effusion of fluid under the skin (oedema). This swelling is soft and 'doughy' and when pressed is not painful, while the depression made by the fingers takes some time to fill up again. The condition worsens over a few hours, the animal becomes acutely ill due to the absorption of toxins, and death may follow in 12–24 hours.

DIAGNOSIS   The disease should always be suspected when a sudden swelling of the head occurs in rams, though a definite conclusion can be reached only after a laboratory examination.

TREATMENT   Immediate and early treatment with black disease serum plus large doses of antibiotic will often result in cure. Your veterinary surgeon should be consulted immediately. However, many combined vaccines contain black disease antigen and such vaccines will prevent the disease.

BLACKQUARTER

CAUSE   Blackquarter results from the invasion of the muscle tissues by a specific group of microbes, the most important of which is *Clostridium chauvoei*. These germs produce resistant, non-active forms known as spores which can live in a dormant state for long periods in the soil. When ingested by the grazing sheep the spores reach the muscle tissue, the liver and other organs where they may remain latent without causing any apparent ill effect unless stirred into virulent activity.

CONDITIONS OF OCCURRENCE   Blackquarter more commonly affects younger animals that are in good, thriving condition. In sheep the disease often occurs after such operations as dipping, docking, castration or vaccination. The reason for this is not yet clearly understood. It may be that the disease results from direct wound infection, but it is also supposed that any undue disturbance—even rough handling—may activate the latent bacterial spores which then multiply and produce their toxins. There is some evidence to suggest that climatic conditions may influence the incidence of the disease. Certainly, if sheep graze on stubble or rough herbage in wet weather, outbreaks are more prevalent, probably because of the greater soil contamination of the feet and muzzle and the increased exposure to the risk of small abrasions. Similarly, when pasture is bare and sheep have of necessity to graze close on soil-contaminated herbage a greater number of spores are likely to be ingested. The disease is usually confined to certain farms and even certain fields and may break out when the animals start to thrive.

SYMPTOMS   The disease may attack any group of muscles but the most commonly affected are those of the legs and back. When a leg is involved the sheep becomes lame, the affected muscle swells, is hot and spongy to the touch and the animal ceases to feed and to ruminate. The course of the disease is usually so short that no illness is observed; the affected sheep is simply found dead. Recovery from blackquarter is very rare, though early treatment with antibiotics has been reported to be useful.

POST-MORTEM FINDINGS   The carcase decomposes rapidly after death. The affected muscle is dark, often blackish-red in colour, and it and its surrounding tissues are infiltrated with a blood-tinged, jelly-like fluid often containing little bubbles of gas. The affected muscle is dry and contains gas.

DIAGNOSIS   A precise diagnosis can be made only by bacteriological examination in the laboratory.

PREVENTION   The incidence of the disease can be largely reduced by vaccination. On pastures where the known incidence has been high, preventive vaccination may be applied, particularly at those times when risk of infection is known to be increased, as at marking time; but on many farms the occurrence of the disease is so sporadic that vaccination is not an economic measure. Again, however, protection against this condition is a common constituent of combined vaccines.

Since the infected carcase contains the spores of the causal microbe it must be buried deeply in quicklime and any contaminated surface soil should be buried with it.

Those fields known to be associated with the occurrence of the disease may be ploughed up and cultivated. This does not, however, preclude the possibility that they will remain infective when, possibly several years later, they are again put under grass.

BRAXY

CAUSE   Braxy, or 'sickness', is due to invasion of the body by a microbe known as *Clostridium septicum*. The disease was blamed for many deaths which were due to pulpy kidney, black disease, etc, and though outbreaks occur, it is not as common as it once was.

CONDITIONS OF OCCURRENCE   Braxy commonly attacks hoggs, especially those in thriving condition. The disease is confined principally to hill grazings and the majority of cases occur in the autumn and winter. Climatic conditions appear to play some considerable part in the production of the disease and the association of the occurrence of braxy with hoar-frost is well recognised.

SYMPTOMS   The course of the disease is so short that affected sheep are usually found dead, but if seen during the short period of observable illness there is considerable swelling of the abdomen, accompanied by signs of abdominal pain.

POST-MORTEM FINDINGS   An inflamed patch on the lining membrane of the fourth stomach is a characteristic lesion. This is the only diagnostic feature on post-mortem examination. Such other lesions as may be present result from acute toxaemia and are common to several diseases. The carcase putrefies rapidly and soon becomes distended with gas.

PREVENTION The infection can be prevented by vaccine and again most combined vaccines contain this antigen and are effective.

The sheep develops a degree of protection some 14 days after vaccination. The inoculation, therefore, should be carried out shortly before the commencement of the seasonal occurrence of the disease. On farms where the disease is virulent it is advisable to vaccinate twice, allowing an interval of one month to elapse between inoculations. Double vaccination is recommended by most producers of vaccine.

Because of a prevalent but erroneous belief that braxy vaccine is in some way detrimental to the hogg it is a common practice to give a dose smaller than that stated on the label of the vaccine container. An effective immunity does not develop if the dose is reduced and the full dose should always be given. Experiments have shown that halving the dose has no beneficial effect and produced no evidence that a check did result from vaccination.

TETANUS (Lockjaw)

Tetanus is an acute nervous disease characterised by continuous, painful spasm of different groups of muscles including those of the jaws ('lockjaw').

CAUSE The cause is a microbe named *Clostridium tetani* which is commonly present in soil enriched with farmyard manure and in small enclosed pastures heavily contaminated with dung. If conditions are favourable, on gaining entrance to a wound, the microbe produces a powerful toxin which is absorbed and on reaching the nerve centres, causes the characteristic spasms.

CONDITIONS OF OCCURRENCE The disease is relatively rare in adult sheep in Britain but it is believed that in lambs infection can occur through the navel. More commonly, infection follows castration and docking, especially if these operations are performed in foul, muddy pens or other such enclosures; rubber rings seem to favour the development of tetanus. Very infrequently tetanus has been observed in the ewe shortly after lambing. From what has been said it will be understood that the disease is more commonly encountered in inbye rather than in hill flocks.

SYMPTOMS In relatively mild cases, apart from dullness and dejection, only a stiff, stilted gait may be observed; the disease may progress no further and if the lamb is nursed and artificially suckled, spontaneous recovery may eventually result. Usually, however, these symptoms quickly develop in intensity and soon the animal is unable to walk or even to stand. The head and neck are often drawn backwards and to one side; the muscles of the trunk and limbs are thrown into intense spasm; the jaws are fixed and the whole animal becomes rigid. The spasms are rendered even more acute by handling the animal or merely tapping the body with the fingers. Death generally results after a very short course of illness, though some animals live for days and may recover if they can swallow.

POST-MORTEM FINDINGS   No characteristic lesions are present. The portal of entry of the microbes, *eg* the unhealed navel, castration and docking wounds, may be found to be suppurative and necrotic.

DIAGNOSIS   The characteristic continuous muscular spasm is in itself diagnostic.

TREATMENT AND PREVENTION   Curative treatment may be attempted only in mild cases. The lamb should be given antibiotics and should be disturbed as little as possible but if it is unable to suck artificial feeding should be introduced. Such measures, however, are seldom of any avail and immediate destruction of the lamb is usually the better course.

The observation of proper care and cleanliness in lambing, castration and docking goes a long way towards preventing occurrences of the disease. Where the disease is provided for in a combined vaccine, lambs will, of course, have some measure of protection.

METRITIS (Inflammation)

This condition occurs in newly-lambed ewes and is usually associated with retention of the afterbirth. Occasionally, however, the disease assumes the proportions of an outbreak and losses can be heavy. Such outbreaks are the result of certain germs gaining entrance to the lambing flock and being transmitted by the lamber's hands and clothing. For this reason lambing hygiene is essential.

CAUSE   The cause is the multiplication of a number of bacteria in the womb especially when the afterbirth is retained. Antibiotic pessaries may be useful in such cases but the treatment can be disappointing. Abortion is a not infrequent prelude to this particular condition.

Certain bacteria of the anaerobic group previously mentioned can cause outbreaks of disease but the use of combined vaccines makes this uncommon. Other organisms which are sometimes involved are *streptococci*, the *corynebacteria*, which are the common pus-producing organisms in sheep and, with increasing frequency, the food poisoning organisms or *salmonellae*.

SYMPTOMS   With organisms other than the anaerobes or gas gangrene bacteria, the symptoms are those of a very sick animal with, usually, a raised temperature and a discharge from the vulva. Death occurs after a few days' illness. The anaerobic infections kill very quickly and are usually accompanied by marked swelling and discolouration of the vulva and of the hairless region under the tail. A blood-stained discharge is common. The anaerobic bacteria concerned are usually *Clostridium oedematiens* and *Clostridium chauvoei*.

DIAGNOSIS   Metritis is easily diagnosed but treatment depends on the identification of the causal organism and laboratory techniques are required for this.

TREATMENT AND PREVENTION   Sporadic instances can be reduced in number by careful hygiene and antibiotic treatment in cases of retained afterbirth. Salmonellae require specific treatment and this is always a matter for the veterinary surgeon. Use of a combined vaccine will prevent the development of the anaerobic form of the disease; where vaccines have not been used, accurate diagnosis will enable a specific serum to be injected in the ewes still to lamb, thus controlling the outbreak. In an emergency, it may be necessary to give antibiotics to every ewe at lambing. In any outbreak it is essential to seek early veterinary and laboratory advice so that the causal organism can be identified and the specific treatment adopted without delay.

COLIBACILLOSIS (Watery Mouth)

This disease has been with us for some time but only in recent years has its association with the bacterium *Escherichia coli* become obvious. This microbe is associated with bowel infections of the newborn in all domestic animals and in man.

CONDITIONS OF OCCURRENCE   There are several factors which play a part in the development of this infection. It rarely appears at the beginning of lambing, but rather as a result of a 'build-up' of infection in lambing fields and more particularly lambing pens, where strains of the organism capable of causing disease become very numerous, with the result that the resistance of the lamb is overcome. Obviously, the more intensive methods of lambing favour the development of the disease. Another important factor is the amount of colostrum or first milk which the lamb gets. This usually contains enough protection to safeguard the lamb against the usual coliform bacteria, but if for any reason it is in short supply, the lamb will be very susceptible to infection.

SYMPTOMS   Diarrhoea or scour is not a constant feature of this disease in the lamb, as it is in other species; this is probably due to the comparative speed with which a lamb succumbs to the infection. Most often the lamb is seen to stop sucking, become dull and sink quite rapidly into a comatose state. In some cases the abdomen is distended. Affected lambs usually die within 12–24 hours of symptoms being noticed. The muzzle is often wet with regurgitated stomach contents—hence the name 'watery mouth'. This latter sign can, however, have other causes, *eg* failure of the bowel to function.

POST-MORTEM FINDINGS   These are usually quite non-specific but in many cases the stomach is distended with fluid, usually milk, but sometimes clear mucoid material, and the succeeding part of the small bowel usually contains more fluid than normal. In many cases the meconium or foetal dung is still present in the coiled large bowel. If the meconium has been voided the lamb will usually have scoured.

DIAGNOSIS   This is dependent on laboratory and bacteriological examination and the elimination of other likely causes of death, of which the most difficult to differentiate are starvation and chilling.

PREVENTION Means of preventing this disease becoming a problem were discussed in the section on lambing pens and housing of ewes (*see* page 3). It is important not to use the same pens from the beginning to the end of lambing. When the disease appears it is obvious that the pens are infected and they should be abandoned if at all possible. If this is not possible then antibiotics, given by mouth as soon after birth as possible and before symptoms develop, can give very good results. As the diagnosis should be made by a veterinary surgeon, in collaboration with a laboratory, he will know the antibiotic to prescribe. One dose given by mouth to each lamb is usually effective.

In 'watery mouth' or 'slavers' caused by retained meconium, laxatives at birth give excellent results.

LIVER NECROSIS

This is a disease of lambs from three days to three weeks old. It is invariably fatal and the areas of dead, white liver tissue are obvious and quite characteristic.

CAUSE The disease is caused by the bacterium *Fusiformis necrophorus* which exists in the rumen and diseased feet of some sheep. It is frequently associated with diseased conditions of the mouth and skin.

CONDITIONS OF OCCURRENCE The bacterium enters the body of the lamb by the navel soon after birth, makes its way to the liver and, occasionally, from there into the lungs. The microbe is much more common where sheep are kept intensively and is rarely seen in hill flocks lambing on the hill. Usually only a few lambs are affected, but where the sheep are crowded, the number affected can be quite serious. Like joint-ill the disease may occur sporadically and because of its slow development may have affected many lambs before its presence is suspected.

SYMPTOMS Symptoms appear three days to three weeks after birth; lambs become listless, tucked up and, in the more chronic cases, may show enlarged abdomens. Death follows 24–72 hours after the symptoms are noticed.

POST-MORTEM FINDINGS Whitish hard areas unlike liver tissue are found in the liver and sometimes in the lungs. These vary in size but may be quite large. There is always quite a sharp line between this area and the more normal liver tissue.

DIAGNOSIS This is a simple matter for the veterinary surgeon and laboratory examination is not necessary in this disease.

PREVENTION Cleanliness is important and sources of infection, such as sheep with infected feet, should not have access to the lambing pens. Dressing the navel and umbilical cord with iodine or other suitable astringent, antiseptic agent is very helpful in preventing this disease. Antibiotics in the form of an aerosol may also be used.

TICK PYAEMIA (Cripples)

Tick pyaemia is an infection of young lambs characterised by abscess formation in the organs and joints.

CAUSE The abscesses are produced by the microbe *staphylococcus*, but though this organism is ubiquitous, tick pyaemia is not. Tick-borne fever appears to play a very important part in allowing the organism to enter the body and establish local infections (abscesses).

CONDITIONS OF OCCURRENCE As the name suggests, the disease is confined to tick-infested areas. Lambs of about 14 days to six weeks old are mainly susceptible, the disease appearing in mid-May and largely disappearing by mid-June. It is assumed that the microbes, which exist on the skin of the ewes and lambs, gain entry by tick bites and in the presence of tick-borne fever are able to set up disease. The incidence varies considerably from year to year, the highest peak being often associated with the onset of a cold spell.

SYMPTOMS Typical symptoms are dullness and progressive debility. Lameness is common and more than one leg may be affected, making it painful and difficult for the lamb to move. Abscesses in the joints and tendon sheaths are readily seen but, in some cases, the abscesses are confined to the liver and other organs and are only found on post-mortem. These abscesses may rupture, discharging thick creamy pus. Abscesses in the spine are not uncommon and produce complete paralysis of the hind limbs even a year after infection has taken place. This paralysis is sometimes mistaken for swayback or for louping-ill.

POST-MORTEM FINDINGS In the majority of cases abscesses in the joints and/or internal organs are readily found. In cases of paralysis removal of the gut and lungs will often show the abscess swelling on the backbone. In some acute cases, however, where the lamb has been found dead, abscesses may not have had time to form and there is nothing to indicate the cause of death: laboratory examination will generally show the presence of *staphylococci* in the blood and organs.

PREVENTION No completely satisfactory method of treating the disease has yet been evolved, though a measure of control has been achieved by double dipping of the lambs. Smearing with anti-tick creams has also given some degree of control. Very long-acting penicillins which release the antibiotic into the bloodstream for up to three weeks after injection have given promising results. These, however, suffer from the disadvantage that the onset of the disease in the flock must be accurately anticipated and the high cost of the drug limits its use to severely affected areas.

TREATMENT This is not very successful though very early treatment with penicillin is likely to save a large proportion of affected lambs.

SPINAL ABSCESS (Paralysis)

This disease has been mentioned under tick pyaemia to which it is a not infrequent sequel. The condition can, however, occur in lambs under all systems of management.

The age most commonly affected is one to three months of age, but occasionally adult sheep show signs of the disease.

SYMPTOMS In the majority of cases, the symptoms are a complete loss of power in the hind limbs, which are dragged, or the animal may assume a 'sitting dog' posture. The animal remains bright and the forelimbs are usually capable of normal movement. In a small number of cases the paralysis is incomplete and the animal is capable of some hind limb movement and is able to stand with assistance.

POST-MORTEM FINDINGS Lesions are confined to the spine in which an abscess will be found, usually behind the withers or in the 'saddle' region. The abscess may vary considerably in size and may not always be easy to find. Usually part of a vertebra is destroyed, the bone being replaced by pus, which forces its way up into the spinal canal resulting in pressure on the spinal cord and paralysis. In young animals *staphylococci* can usually be cultured from this pus, but organisms are absent in older animals indicating that the lesion is long-standing. It is believed that all such infections take place early in life, but should the lesion become quiescent, paralysis will occur only when the vertebrae is subjected to strain, *eg* fighting in rams.

In rare cases the abscess may be nearer the brain causing all four limbs to be affected.

CONTROL There is no specific control measure but hygiene measures to reduce navel infection are recommended.

JOINT-ILL

CAUSE Joint-ill in lambs results from infection at, or soon after, birth by certain microbes which, in the majority of cases, are pus-forming *streptococci*. A specific infection—Erysipelas (*see* page 29)—also occurs.

CONDITIONS OF OCCURRENCE The disease arises from the infection of exposed surfaces such as the navel and the wounds resulting from docking and castration. The incidence is usually highest when lambing has been carried out in small, enclosed fields or paddocks since these can become heavily contaminated with the causal microbes. Obviously, an infected lambing pen is even more dangerous.

SYMPTOMS The primary symptoms usually observed are dullness and loss of appetite quickly followed by the sudden appearance of swelling, accompanied by tenderness and pain, in one or more of the joints of the legs. As the swelling progressively increases the lamb becomes less active and may even be completely immobilised. The enlarged joint may rupture and discharge a considerable quantity of pus.

POST-MORTEM FINDINGS On post-mortem examination the affected joints and tendon sheaths are found to contain pus and erosions of the joint surfaces may be present.

DIAGNOSIS It is always advisable to have the type of infecting microbe identified by a laboratory test, as treatment depends to some extent upon the micro-organism concerned.

TREATMENT The general principles of preventive treatment are those of cleanliness. It should be emphasised that infection can be readily conveyed from lamb to lamb, and the disinfection of hands, etc, should therefore be scrupulously observed by the lambing shepherd.

In affected flocks the application of an astringent, antiseptic dressing to the navel at birth is of value. A 10 per cent solution of copper sulphate is a simple and usually effective application for this purpose; iodine is also effective.

The use of sulpha drugs and penicillin has given encouraging results in the streptococcal form of the disease, but it is essential to the success of these methods of treatment that the nature of the disease be diagnosed as early as possible, as once the pus forms in the joints, treatment is much less effective.

ERYSIPELAS INFECTION: Crippling or Arthritis (Stiff Lamb Disease)

CAUSE This disease results from a chronic inflammation of the joints of the legs by infection with a germ called *Erysipelothrix rhusiopathiae* which is similar, if not identical, to that causing erysipelas in pigs. The germ lives in a certain type of soil, so some farms and even some fields give rise to infection, while the disease is never seen on others. There is, however, no association with pigs, the disease occurring on hill ground as well as in fields.

CONDITIONS OF OCCURRENCE The disease is seen in two forms. The less common is seen in lambs ten days to three weeks of age and is fairly acute, with swelling and fluid in the joints. The course of this form of the disease is similar to that described under joint-ill of which it is, of course, a particular type. The more usual form affects lambs one to six months old and is usually chronic. Infection may result from contaminated docking and castration wounds, which emphasises the need for cleanliness and boiling of instruments used in these operations. However, outbreaks do occur where no wounds have been inflicted. The disease occurs both on inbye and hill ground, though it is rather rare on the hill. The percentage of lambs attacked appears to be related to the intensity of stocking; 5 per cent to 10 per cent of the lambs are frequently affected but higher numbers do occur.

SYMPTOMS   In the early acute form in the younger lambs, swelling of one or more joints and marked lameness are symptoms shared with any type of joint infection and laboratory examination is necessary to diagnose the disease. In the chronic type the onset may be insidious and the disease well-established before it is noticed. In some cases, quite severe lameness is noted early on, but often a gradual stiffening and failure to thrive is observed. In many cases, when the disease has been present for some weeks, there is twisting or distortion of the joint or joints. Swelling of the joints is not common in this form, though puffiness and excess fluid can often be detected on close examination. The disease is prolonged and affected lambs are underdeveloped and ill-thriven. The disease is rarely fatal, though deaths may result from intercurrent disease, *eg* pneumonia and parasitism, which commonly affect chronically sick sheep. Occasionally the valves of the heart are attacked and death in such cases is sudden.

POST-MORTEM FINDINGS   These are not very noticeable to the untrained eye but the joint membranes are thickened and there are ulcers on the joint surfaces. The joint fluid is thick and may contain little rice grain-like bodies but pus is absent.

DIAGNOSIS   While the general history of the affected lambs strongly indicates erysipelas, laboratory confirmation is necessary.

TREATMENT   Once the disease is well established treatment is of little avail because of the joint damage and the difficulty of killing the organisms in the joint. In early cases, however, penicillin is valuable and the use of antiserum may prevent the spread to the unaffected lambs.

PREVENTION   In those cases where the disease occurs annually in younger lambs, vaccination of the ewes with swine erysipelas vaccine before lambing has given promising results, The same advice as is given for the control of colibacillosis and joint-ill (*see* pages 25 and 28) will, however, if rigorously applied, greatly reduce the incidence of the disease. Instruments used in cutting and docking should be cleaned and disinfected or sterilised at regular intervals throughout the proceedings, and if the disease has been occurring regularly, the operations should be carried out in temporary pens well away from the permanent pens which may be heavily infected. Any unusually high incidence of crippling should be referred at once to a veterinary surgeon.

FOOT-ROT

The term 'foot-rot of sheep' has been loosely applied to any diseased condition of the feet that is associated with lameness; but here the term is understood as relating to a specific contagious disease, resulting from the invasion of the soft, sensitive structures of the foot by certain microbes.

CAUSE   The microbes concerned, of which the most important is believed to be an organism named *Fusiformis nodosus*, can remain inactive but potentially dangerous in cracks and crevices of the foot for prolonged periods—at least nine months—but if removed from the feet of sheep they cannot survive for longer than seven days. These microbes attack only the sheep and goat and no other animal.

Conditions of Occurrence   Sheep of all ages are susceptible. Conditions in which the feet tend to become sodden and soft—prolonged wet weather and enclosed, badly-drained, rank pastures—predispose to infection but the disease will not occur on such pastures unless the specific microbes are present.

Symptoms   Commonly the first sign of foot-rot is observed in the sudden occurrence of lameness among several members of a flock at about the same time. The disease usually begins as a mild inflammation of the soft tissues between the horny hooves. The skin covering these tissues breaks and infection enters and progresses under the horny wall and the sole, which become separated from the underlying sensitive structures by suppurative evil-smelling material.

The extent of the diseased area varies considerably, but in neglected cases the horn of the whole hoof may be under-run by the infection. Two or more feet are usually affected and the lameness may be so severe that when the fore feet are involved grazing is possible only if the sheep assumes a kneeling position. When other feet are also affected, grazing may become impossible and the consequent loss of physical condition may be rapid.

Diagnosis   Lameness in individual members of a flock may arise from accidental injury and also from other causes, but the occurrence of lameness in several sheep at about the same time should raise the suspicion of the presence of foot-rot. The possibility of foot-and-mouth disease must, however, be remembered. In any case, a close examination is called for since the characteristic nature of the disease is usually readily apparent.

Foot-soreness due to travelling long distances over hard roads is usually readily recognised. In contagious pustular dermatitis (orf) the region of the coronet is often the site of the lesions, but the hoof itself is not involved. Outbreaks of foot-and-mouth disease have been mistaken for those of foot-rot. In nearly all such cases it has been found that a close examination of the feet had not been carried out.

Curative Treatment   In dealing with outbreaks of foot-rot the following three facts must be kept in mind:
(1) The disease is due to the attack of a specific microbe.
(2) The microbes concerned can be harboured in the feet for several months.
(3) The microbes, if removed from the feet of the sheep, cannot live on pastures, etc, for more than seven days.

Based on these considerations treatment should proceed on the following lines:
(a)   The feet of each member of the whole flock should be carefully examined and the diseased cases separated from those that are not apparently affected. This examination necessitates the turning of every sheep and gentle paring with a knife. The unaffected sheep should be passed very slowly through a foot-trough containing an 8–10 per cent solution of formalin (about half a pint of formalin

to each gallon of water), after which they should be placed in a clean, uncontaminated pasture, *ie* a pasture which has been free from sheep for at least 14 days.

Subsequently, the sheep should be passed through the foot-bath two or three times at intervals of about ten days and should not be returned to their original pasture until after the lapse of a month to ensure that they are no longer carriers of the specific germs. During this quarantine period they should also be periodically examined for any early signs of the disease.

(*b*) The obviously affected cases must be treated individually by having the horn of each diseased foot pared and trimmed and the greyish-yellow diseased tissue removed before further treatment is applied. It is important to remember that the wall of the hoof as well as the sole requires attention.

This 'paring and trimming' is often lightly regarded, as if it were a simple and easy matter requiring little experience or particular care. In point of fact, such procedure on a diseased foot constitutes a surgical operation requiring skill and understanding. While each individual case should be treated in respect of the conditions present, the dead and separating horn should be pared off by the knife or by secateurs to expose the diseased tissue. Ignorant and unskilful persons tend to remove not only the diseased material but also much healthy tissue, thus not only maiming the animal by causing serious damage to the foot, but also inflicting much needless pain and suffering. The operator should try to avoid causing bleeding as this obscures the field of operation and indicates that healthy tissue has been damaged. This is not always easy and if bleeding starts, no more paring should be done and the foot should be treated with an antibiotic aerosol or another effective preparation prescribed by a veterinary surgeon. Treating with antibiotics should also follow where the lesions are extensive and severe and where it is impossible on humane grounds to finish the operation in one attempt. Such sheep should be retained in a paddock for a day or two before completing the paring, treatment being administered every three days if necessary. The reason for using antibiotics is to provide protection without hardening of the hoof which makes further paring difficult, if not impossible.

In other less severe cases, where all under-run horn has been successfully pared away, the foot should be immersed in a jar of 6–7 per cent formalin for about a minute. The affected animals should then be passed through the foot bath and pastured separately from the clean sheep till they can be examined at 7 and at 14 days to ensure that there has been no recurrence of the disease. They can then be returned to the healthy flock. When examining feet after the first treatment, be sure to put the healthiest sheep through the pens first, finishing with those most likely to be infected. In very advanced, neglected cases, in which the feet are deformed, it is more economical and safer to have the animals slaughtered.

It must be emphasised that only relatively mild preparations should be used on diseased feet. The application of strong caustic chemicals cannot be too strongly condemned for such substances destroy the healthy tissue and hinder, rather than encourage, healing.

PREVENTIVE TREATMENT (1) It is advisable to keep infected pastures, pens, etc free of sheep for 14 days by which time the infective agent will have perished.

(2) It is much more difficult to clear the infection from diseased sheep than to destroy it on the land, and sheep which have been under treatment should not be returned to the main flock until it is certain that a complete cure has been effected.

(3) The shepherd's instruments and his hands should be washed and disinfected after each sheep has been dressed, and horn parings, infected dressings, etc should be collected and destroyed.

(4) Sheep that are obviously affected should not be passed through the foot-bath or placed in pens immediately before these are used by the apparently healthy members of the flock.

(5) Newly purchased sheep should be carefully examined for the presence of foot-rot and, even if apparently healthy, should be passed through the foot-bath. They should be kept by themselves for at least two weeks, after which, if there is no sign of disease, they may be introduced into the general area of clean land.

From what has been said it will be apparent that once a flock is free from foot-rot it can be kept free. The procedure, though laborious and by no means simple, is rewarding when freedom from the disease is achieved.

FOOT ABSCESS

CAUSE The condition results from infection of the joint above the clit. If the abscess has not burst, the joint and/or the tissues around the joint are found to contain dark watery evil-smelling pus. When a channel to the outside forms, however, organisms which then gain entrance produce thick whitish pus. The original infection appears to be *Fusiformis necrophorus*, though the pus is often sterile when examined in the laboratory.

SYMPTOMS The first sign is that of lameness in one foot—usually a forefoot. The coronet swells steadily and the two clits become widely separated, the sheep refusing to put the affected foot to the ground. Later, pus starts to discharge from one or two small holes above the coronet. Prior to this there is rarely any external sign of disease on the coronet itself.

COURSE OF THE CONDITION In those cases where the joint itself is not involved healing occasionally takes place after rupture, but this is rare. Most cases continue to discharge and the animal loses condition. Death from pneumonia may follow, but generally the animal is slaughtered before this.

TREATMENT As the bone is so frequently damaged, antibiotic treatment is effective in a small proportion of cases only. Where valuable breeding stock is affected, the infected digit can be removed surgically by a veterinary surgeon.

SCAD (Scald)

This disease is a bacterial infection of the skin between the clits and in the bulb of the heel.

CAUSE   Bacteria isolated from the lesion include corynebacteria and *Fusiformis necrophorus*. An organism resembling *Fusiformis nodosus*—the cause of foot-rot—has been described in Australia. *Fusiformis necrophorus* is certainly associated with some outbreaks of this type of disease in Scotland, but in view of the fact that more than one organism seems capable of infecting this area in the sheep, the name and symptoms may cover more than one type of infection.

CONDITIONS OF OCCURRENCE   The disease is most often seen in late summer, particularly in wet years, and is most common amongst lambs. There is considerable variation in virulence and while in some cases only a few lambs may be affected, in others, the majority may be lame in one or more feet and the ewes may also show the effects of the disease. On occasion ewes may suffer an outbreak in winter, so the disease cannot be regarded as seasonal.

SYMPTOMS   Lameness is the first and indeed the only sign in the affected flock. On closer examination the skin between the clits will be found to be swollen, white and denuded of hair and with an offensive smell. The lesion may be confined to the part between the heels but may extend to all the interdigital skin. In very severe cases some separation of horn may be observed. The condition is often extremely painful and when more than one foot is affected the animal is reluctant to move and may lose condition.

COURSE OF THE DISEASE   Lesions usually heal in two to three weeks, but other feet may become infected in turn. The condition can remain in the flock for two months or more if not treated.

TREATMENT   This condition responds well to early treatment. Rather caustic pastes were once popular but it is now generally recognised that less damaging medicaments are preferable. Good results can be obtained by treating all clinically affected feet with antibiotic, either in the form of an ointment or an aerosol. The remaining sheep are passed slowly through a footbath containing 5 per cent formalin. The animals should then be returned to a clean pasture and the treatment repeated in one week. The affected pasture should be rested for 14 days.

There is no known preventive treatment.

JOHNE'S DISEASE (Paratuberculosis)

Johne's Disease in sheep is a specific bacterial infection of the intestine and its associated lymph glands. The disease is chronic in type and in its advanced stages is characterised by progressive loss of bodily condition and general debility.

CAUSE   The cause is a microbe known as Johne's bacillus. In some cases the bacilli which infect sheep are identical with those that also cause Johne's disease in cattle, but in other cases the bacilli concerned would appear to belong to strains peculiar to the sheep.

CONDITIONS OF OCCURRENCE Infection results from the ingestion of the microbes on infected pastures and probably occurs early in lamb-hood, although the symptoms rarely manifest themselves until the sheep is about two years of age. This is because the incubation period is prolonged (it may be one year or more) and also because the bacilli appear to be activated by the stress of pregnancy and lactation. Thus, pregnant gimmers, or ewes with their first lambs at foot, are those in which the disease is most commonly observed. Adult sheep are relatively resistant to infection.

Pastures become infected by the deposit of the microbes excreted in the droppings by infected animals. The length of time that pastures vacated by infective animals remain infected is not known, but pasture-infection persists certainly for several months; possibly for one year or even longer.

Although the whole flock has been exposed to infection, usually only a relatively small number of the sheep become diseased.

SYMPTOMS The disease is indicated by progressive weakness and emaciation (pine). In odd cases an intermittent scour may occur but this is unusual, and the animal may even be constipated. Anaemia is always evident, especially in the later stages of the disease; dropsical swellings may appear, particularly under the lower jaw, but this is rare. The sheep, in general, presents an unthrifty appearance; the fleece lacks lustre, is broken and ragged and pulls out readily on handling.

POST-MORTEM FINDINGS The signs of emaciation are usually obvious; the body-fat may disappear and be replaced by a gelatinous material. The lining membrane of the small intestine, particularly that of its terminal portion, is much thickened and solid in consistence; its surface may show cracks and corrugations and is sometimes yellow in colour. In advanced cases the caecum and large intestine may also be involved. The associated lymph glands are enlarged and their lymphatic vessels are corded.

While these changes occur in typical cases, in others there may be no apparent thickening of the bowel wall and its lining membrane may not show any obvious signs of disease. The glands, however, are usually enlarged.

DIAGNOSIS Symptoms of progressive weakness and emaciation, without diarrhoea, in isolated cases in gimmers or young ewes are suspicious signs of Johne's disease. Some forms of worm and fluke infestation give rather similar symptoms but usually more ewes are affected. Worm egg counts are not of much value in differentiating the infection, for ewes with Johne's disease may also have worms. The presence of fluke eggs in numbers does, of course, confirm this condition.

The symptoms of cobalt deficiency pine (*see* page 57) to some extent simulate those of Johne's disease, but in cobalt pine there is a history of annual recurrence over a long period of years and again many animals are affected—often the hoggs. In pine, recovery takes place on treatment.

Diagnosis may be established in the laboratory by demonstrating the causal organism in the dung. Failure to demonstrate the microbes does not, however, exclude the possibility of Johne's disease, and a reliable diagnosis may only be made on post-mortem examination of one or more of the affected animals.

Specific diagnostic tests by the use of johnin (paratuberculin) and the complement fixation test have not yet proved reliable.

PREVENTION   There is no known cure for the disease, but its incidence may be reduced considerably in affected flocks by the immediate slaughter of obvious cases, thus decreasing the level of infection on the pastures. In severely infected flocks vaccination gives good results.

The progress of the disease is so slow and insidious that it often becomes established in a flock and the pastures become infected before its presence is realised.

Since lambs are most susceptible to infection, the apparently healthy ewes and their lambs should, under veterinary supervision, be separated from suspected cases and removed from the infected pastures.

Where practicable, all lambs raised on infected pastures should be fattened and sold and not used for breeding.

Infective pastures should, where possible, be ploughed and cultivated before being again used by sheep. Should this be impracticable the contaminated pasture should be kept free of sheep for at least 12 months and, when sheep are next introduced to it, only adult animals should be grazed.

It will be apparent from what has been written that the cause of Johne's disease in sheep is quite definitely known and the way by which these animals contract and, in turn, transmit the infection is largely understood: but a specific test by which its presence in the sheep can be definitely determined has not been developed, though vaccination is a feasible and useful preventive in the rare flock where infection is heavy.

ACTINOBACILLOSIS (Cruels; Grothels)

Actinobacillosis in sheep is characterised by chronic abscess formation of the tissues of the head, lungs and also of the lymphatic system. The incidence of this disease is relatively low but since it attacks rams it is of considerable importance.

CAUSE   The cause is a microbe known as *Actinobacillus lignieresi* which is indistinguishable from the organism that causes 'wooden tongue' in cattle.

CONDITIONS OF OCCURRENCE   Infection gains entrance to the body in wounds and abrasions of the skin, particularly on the lips which are usually the first tissues affected. Its relative frequency in rams has been attributed to injury following fighting, in which case the primary site of infection may be the base of the horn. The disease is usually seen only in adults but occasionally younger animals are affected.

SYMPTOMS   The disease almost invariably starts on the head, swelling of the lips being the earliest sign. Later, lumps appear on the cheeks, the jaw and the glands of the neck. The swellings slowly increase in size to about that of a walnut or larger and become the seat of multiple abscesses which may burst and discharge a small quantity of yellowish-green or greyish-green, sticky pus. Later, healing of the abscesses may leave thick, hairless scars. Other abscesses form in the adjacent tissue and the diseased area becomes widespread, seriously interfering with feeding and rumination and even rendering these impossible. Until this stage is reached, however, the general body condition is well maintained.

Involvement of internal organs, *eg* the lungs, is not known to give rise to recognisable symptoms, but rams are occasionally subject to infection of the penis and prepuce (sheath). The affected organs are swollen and discoloured and a purulent discharge is emitted. This condition may seriously interfere with urination.

POST-MORTEM FINDINGS On dissecting the head, multiple thick-walled abscesses are present in the soft tissues and commonly involve the bones of the jaws and face; they contain the characteristic greenish, thick, sticky pus.

When the lungs are affected the lesions are those of multiple abscesses which commonly range from a pea to a hazel nut in size and contain the characteristic pus. The surrounding lung tissue is usually unaffected. Similar lesions may be present, though more rarely, in the liver and kidneys and also in the body lymph glands, particularly at the point of the shoulder.

TREATMENT Removal of isolated abscesses and drainage of larger abscesses can be helpful, while the injection of sodium iodide is reported to give good results in early cases. However, one antibiotic preparation which must, of course, be administered by a veterinary surgeon, shows considerable promise.

LISTERIOSIS (Circling Disease)

Listeriosis is an infectious disease to which many species, including man, are subject. It affects brain tissue and also causes abortion.

CAUSE The cause is infection by the microbe *Listeria monocytogenes*.

CONDITIONS OF OCCURRENCE The organism can live in the soil, manure and silage for many months and infection probably results from ingestion. Silage feeding has been blamed on more than one occasion. It is not common in Scotland but sporadic cases do occur and in view of its being harmful to man it is important to treat possible cases with care.

SYMPTOMS The organisms may cause abortion without other signs in the ewe. In the lamb it causes acute disease, with death following a day or so after symptoms, which are vague and of little diagnostic value, are noticed. The type of disease most commonly seen is that which occurs in the ewe when infection enters the brain. The animal ceases to feed and there may be a discharge from nose and eyes. Commonly, one ear droops, the head is drawn to one side and the animal moves in a circle, always in the same direction. The disease may progress rapidly and the animal will go down in two to three days with death occurring within a week. In other cases the duration is longer, with the tendency to circle the only noticeable symptom.

DIAGNOSIS Laboratory examination is necessary to determine this organism as the cause of abortion. In the lamb the characteristic 'sawdust' appearance of the liver due to myriads of tiny abscesses is rather characteristic, but laboratory confirmation is necessary. In older animals the signs are difficult to differentiate from gid or an abscess in the brain. These can, of course, be eliminated by visual examination of the brain itself, but a microscopic examination is necessary to confirm listeriosis.

TREATMENT AND PREVENTION There is no effective treatment and as cases in an adult flock rarely exceed three to four animals prevention does not appear important. In lambs, however, the appearance of the disease means that the infected pens must be closed and the ewes still to lamb moved to clean ground.

ACUTE OR GANGRENOUS MASTITIS (Udderclap)

CAUSE Acute mastitis or inflammation of the udder, commonly known as 'udderclap', is produced by a number of pus-forming organisms, the most common being *staphylococci*. Organisms of the pasteurella group, and the common cause of suppuration in the sheep—*corynebacterium pyogenes*—are, however, sometimes involved.

CONDITIONS OF OCCURRENCE Though occasionally the incidence is high, generally only a small number of ewes is affected in any one flock. The disease is most common in the six weeks after lambing; a lamb with orf (*see* page 50) will transmit that disease to the udder and teats of the ewe, in which case, the development of acute mastitis is very probable. The disease is more prevalent in the heavier milking, lowground sheep than in hill breeds. Cases often appear to follow cold spells and chilling of the udder is commonly believed to be a contributory factor. Certainly, injuries are important as points of entry for the causal germs, which are widespread and, given suitable conditions, will invade the udder and set up disease.

SYMPTOMS The first sign observed is a slight limp, caused by the ewe carrying a leg wide to favour the affected teat. The affected half of the udder becomes swollen and inflamed and within a few hours an acute toxic condition develops from which the ewe may die. The affected udder may become gangrenous (cold and dark purple in colour) before death occurs. In less acute cases the ewe survives, though the affected portion of the udder may slough off or become hard and useless.

DIAGNOSIS Diagnosis is simple on examination of the udder but early recognition of the limp as a symptom of this disease is important.

PREVENTION There is no effective method of prevention; control of orf is, however, one way of avoiding heavy losses.

TREATMENT Very early treatment with antibiotics, both into the teat canal and by injection, is of value and will often cut short an attack. Once the disease is established, the affected half will invariably be destroyed. Treatment with antibiotics and, if necessary, veterinary surgical treatment, can save the lives of the ewes.

CHRONIC MASTITIS

CAUSE Various microbes have been recovered from udders showing lesions of this disease but, as in gangrenous mastitis, *Staphylococcus aureus* is the most common. Predisposing causes, *eg* overstocking of the udder after weaning, are regarded as favouring this disease.

CONDITIONS OF OCCURRENCE This form of mastitis is common in the North Country Cheviot breed and an incidence of up to 10 per cent, and occasionally even higher, has been recorded. The mortality rate is low, but because they would be unable to rear twins, affected ewes have to be discarded and this can represent a heavy financial loss. The disease, which may be found in ewes of any age and in gimmers, is essentially a post-weaning condition, although cases may sometimes arise prior to weaning. The first month after weaning is critical but cases may occur at any time during the dry period.

SYMPTOMS A badly affected ewe may be seen dragging a hind leg, but most cases are not discovered until the sheep is turned up and the udder examined. An acute phase may take place without any noticeable clinical signs. The lesions, which can apparently develop within a few days, are not a sequel to gangrenous mastitis, although the latter may occur in the same flock. In many cases no abnormality is noticed till the ewes lamb the following spring, when one half of the udder is found to have withered and to be completely useless. Occasionally, when some milk is being produced, a hard cord can be felt blocking the teat.

In a typical case one half of the udder becomes swollen and hard (fibrosis). Large nodules or lumps (abscesses) may protrude from the surface of the udder and after an abscess has come to a head, thick pus escapes. It may or may not be possible to draw pus from the udder via the teat. In other cases, smaller nodules may be felt near the base of one or both teats which are often found to be 'blind'. In every instance lesions tend to contract over a period but milk secretion is lost and the ewe is of no further value for breeding.

DIAGNOSIS The lesions are obvious when the udder is examined. The condition may be suspected when a ewe or gimmer appears to be lame in the post-weaning period.

PREVENTION Management is important. After weaning, ewes should be put on bare pasture to diminish milk production and reduce overstocking of the udder. A laxative may also be helpful for this purpose. In former times it was the custom in many North Country Cheviot flocks to milk out the ewes once, twice, or more frequently, at intervals during the first fortnight after weaning; alternatively, the lambs might be allowed back to suckle at two and five days. Mastitis is said to have been less common then but, of course, other factors may have to be taken into consideration to explain the difference in incidence. If stripping out is attempted, aseptic precautions must be taken to avoid any spread of infection from udder to udder.

The use of antibiotics introduced via the teat in the immediate post-weaning period has been shown to be of some value, but the cost must be taken into account. Post-weaning application of collodion to the teats to form a seal around the teat orifice and prevent entry of infection is claimed to be useful and has the advantage of being cheap. Vaccines have proved to be of no value.

TREATMENT   In the chronic disease when the udder is hard and pockets of pus are present treatment is of no avail.

PNEUMONIA

This disease is one of the most common in sheep. Animals of all ages can be affected and it is frequently the cause of death in animals debilitated by other conditions.

CAUSE   The cause of outbreaks of the disease is still rather obscure though there is some evidence that viruses as well as the common microbe *Pasteurella haemolytica* may be involved. In other cases it results from lungworm infection, abscesses due to *corynebacterium pyogenes* and *staphylococci*, though these latter are usually secondary to conditions such as jaagsieckte, orf, inhalation of medicine, and even tick pyaemia. They are, therefore, of less importance but must be considered when lesions of pneumonia are found in the lungs.

CONDITIONS OF OCCURRENCE   Outbreaks are most common in the spring and early summer months and the factors which trigger them off are difficult to determine, ranging as they do from such widely divergent apparent causes as bringing hill ewes inbye to lamb, to the introduction of too much barley in the feed. In many cases no definite causal factor can be incriminated.

Pneumonia of one lobe of the lung is quite commonly found at the slaughterhouse in fat lambs which were not suspected of having any illness. It is therefore unwise to regard small areas of pneumonia as of great significance. These pneumonic areas are usually of fairly long standing and quiescent. In some cases, however, when animals are moved by road or driven, the condition may flare up and one finds the area of old pneumonia complicated by a recent acute area of infection. Such breakdowns can rapidly result in the death of the animal.

Young lambs of two or three days of age are sometimes affected by the disease, even on the hill, with all the characters of an acute infectious disease. In such cases a particular strain of *Pasteurella haemolytica* is usually isolated and is believed to be the cause. Viruses cannot, however, be ruled out. Tick-borne fever may be a predisposing cause in some outbreaks.

In ewes the condition is particularly prevalent in cast blackface ewes on low ground and is in some way tied up with nutrition and environment. In all flocks, of course, isolated losses from pneumonia occur, but the disease is only of importance when an epidemic occurs.

In the late summer and autumn outbreaks of both chronic pneumonia and a peracute pneumonia are seen in hoggs. These result from very different circumstances. The first—the chronic type—is seen in poorer lambs which are often wormy and not infrequently infested with lungworm as well.

The second peracute type occurs in lambs in varying condition when they are moved from poorish pasture to stubble, particularly barley stubble. This type of change may result in pulpy kidney disease which is often blamed for the losses, as is braxy, since the deaths occur after such a short period of illness as to merit the description of 'sudden'. In many such cases a strain of *Pasteurella haemolytica* can be isolated from every organ in the body—a bacteraemia—with the lungs extremely congested and microscopically showing signs of early widespread pneumonia.

Between these two extremes many outbreaks of severe pneumonia occur, particularly in feeding hoggs.

SYMPTOMS   As already mentioned the disease may vary from sudden death to infection undetected till slaughter. Symptoms do therefore vary and only in acute and subacute cases are they clinically noticeable. The most noticeable feature is difficulty in breathing when being chased or driven. This 'heaving' is, however, also seen in anaemia caused, for example, by fluke, and in jaagsieckte which is often mistaken for pneumonia. Coughing is a common sign and when much coughing is present in the flock on exertion some degree of pneumonia should be suspected. All acute cases show a marked fever. More chronic cases may or may not cough but become ill-thriven and obviously unfit.

POST-MORTEM FINDINGS   The appearance of the affected lungs varies considerably with the type of pneumonia present. The diagnosis of this disease is not always so simple as might be thought and it is surprising how often discolouration and congestion is diagnosed as pneumonia by the layman.

PERACUTE TYPE   Here the lungs, instead of collapsing when the chest is opened, remain prominent and often show the depressions caused by the ribs on their surface. They are dark red, mottled, with slatey blue patches and when cut in the recently dead animal bleed very freely. The air passages contain a frothy, mucoid and often blood-stained exudate. In one less common form the lobules of the lung are very prominent because of the divisions between them becoming swollen with fluid. The lung feels firm and rubbery.

LESS ACUTE TYPE   In this type the front lobes of the lung are definitely solid and liver-like and this may extend to other parts of the lung. The affected and unaffected parts are usually separated by a definite line. In both the types described there may be a varying amount of clear fluid between the lung and the chest wall and sometimes the lung is stuck to the chest wall by a whitish clot of fibrinous material.

DIAGNOSIS The existence of the condition is readily determined by post-mortem examination by a veterinary surgeon. Perhaps what is most important in the presence of the disease is to determine the likely precipitating factor, since the most rational means of arresting it is to remove this cause.

TREATMENT AND PREVENTION Outbreaks of acute pneumonia in feeding lambs and hoggs can be arrested by a change to poorer pasture. A check will often have the same effect, *eg* penning for a day. Where the condition is associated with acidosis and insufficient roughage intake, the answer is obvious. On occasion, however, the identification of the underlying management and environmental factors may be difficult.

In ewes, particularly cast blackface ewes on good pasture, removal to any rough pasture is often effective. Specific vaccines are available and in experimental work have been shown to produce a degree of immunity. They cannot, of course, be expected to protect against all forms of pneumonia and a disease which is so obviously strongly influenced by factors other than simple infection is not ideal for vaccinal protection.

Individual cases can often be successfully treated by antibiotic therapy, but this is definitely a matter for prescription by the veterinary surgeon.

MYCOTIC DERMATITIS

This condition was described in Australia 40 years ago but it is only in the last 10 years that it has been widely recognised in Britain.

CAUSE The cause is an organism which causes skin disease in other species as well as sheep and is referred to variously as *actinomyces dermatonomus*, *actinomyces congolense* and *Dermatophilus*.

CONDITIONS OF OCCURRENCE The condition affects all woolly parts of the body but is most common on the back and sides. The organism invades the roots of the wool causing pustules and exudation. These form a crust which builds up, then becomes very hard, matting the wool fibres together. The scab later separates from the skin but remains in the wool. The disease may not be noticed till the animals are clipped and then the distance of the scab from the skin indicates how long a period has elapsed since infection. Such wool may be downgraded; hence the economic importance of the disease. It is believed that wet seasons favour its development. Lesions have been described on the legs resembling orf and referred to as 'strawberry foot rot'.

SYMPTOMS These are minimal, as only occasional animals show signs of irritation. However, in an infected flock some animals will usually show scabbing on the hair-covered parts of the body—often the ears and the face. This is most common in lambs. In a small number of sheep in an infected flock there will be some wool loss, but though as many as 75 per cent of the animals may be infected, the disease is quite commonly overlooked. Once the existence of the disease is realised, however, affected sheep can often be identified by the appearance of the fleece. When the fleece is parted, varying amounts of wool are seen to be matted together by a scab which varies in colour, being lighter close to the skin.

When sheep are infected experimentally on a small area of skin from which the hair has been plucked, the hair follicles become infected and pustules form within 48 hours. The scab hardens to a crust and separates from the skin in seven to eight days. This same pattern is probably followed in natural infection. This characteristic, which differs from orf, is used in laboratory differentiation of the two diseases.

DIAGNOSIS The disease should be suspected when dark scabs are found matting the wool at various levels, or when hard scabs are felt on the skin of the sheep. The disease requires laboratory confirmation and this is done by examination of the scabs. The results are more reliable when the scab is removed from, or close to, the skin. Soft sebaceous or waxy material sometimes mats the wool, especially in attacks of wool rot, and the disease should be differentiated from this much milder condition.

PREVENTION AND TREATMENT This has not been notably successful in the past but dips and dusting powders specifically formulated to control the condition are now available. It is, however, very important to follow the maker's instructions if satisfactory results are to be achieved.

Individual severely affected sheep can be treated with antibiotics and skin dressings.

FLEECE ROT (Canary Wool; Green Wool)

This condition appears to have become more common in recent years and recognition of the condition may be due in part to the interest in mycotic dermatitis (see page 42) which affects the price given for the wool. Modern dips may also have favoured the development of the condition.

SYMPTOMS The areas most commonly affected are over the back and rump of the sheep. In early stages the wool looks wet and is soapy to the feel, with a rather rancid odour. Discolouration follows, ranging from a dingy brownish shade to intense yellow and green, the colour depending on the bacteria or fungi involved. Later, the condition dries up and the dried material mats the wool fibres; the condition is then easily confused with mycotic dermatitis. While in the active state, wool rot seems attractive to the blowfly and maggoting is often the first thing to attract attention.

TREATMENT The condition responds well to clipping the affected parts when these are small in extent and applying an approved disinfectant ointment or—in more extensive areas—sprays. The condition is controlled to some extent by dips to which the manufacturer has added antiseptics.

INOCULATION SEPSIS (Vaccination Blackquarter)

The disease is the result of the introduction of virulent microbes beneath the skin when giving sheep injections.

CAUSE   The organisms causing the disease are most usually *Corynebacterium pyogenes*—the common pus-forming microbe in the sheep—together with *streptococci*. In some cases the organism of braxy—*Clostridium septicum*—or the one causing blackquarter, *Clostridium chauvoei*, are incriminated. More rarely the black disease microbe, *Clostridium oedematiens*, is introduced.

CONDITIONS OF OCCURRENCE   The disease, as the name implies, follows the administration of vaccines, sera or other medicament by hypodermic injection and results from neglect of the precautions outlined in the section dealing with this subject. Usually the infection is introduced into a bottle of vaccine by a contaminated needle and all the animals subsequently injected from that bottle are affected. In some cases roughness in the use of the syringe, resulting in damaged tissue, is the cause. Bacteria which are introduced are usually overcome by the body defences, but if tissue is torn and damaged, infection is readily established.

SYMPTOMS   When the *Clostridia* mentioned are the cause, the animals can die within a few hours without ever being seen to be ill. With *Corynebacterium* the animals are seen to be lame, with the leg near the site of the injection—usually a foreleg—swollen and puffy. The animals die within one to three days.

POST-MORTEM FINDINGS   These are usually confined to the tissues just beneath the skin, which are waterlogged with a blood-stained fluid which may have the rather characteristic smell associated with the affecting organism, *eg Clostridium septicum* or *Corynebacterium pyogenes*. If the needle has been inserted too deeply, muscle, and even the body cavities, may be infected.

TREATMENT   While massive doses of penicillin given when the first signs of lameness are seen may result in a cure, the success rate is not high. Where a limited number of sheep are involved it may be worthwhile giving a long-acting penicillin to the others without waiting for symptoms to develop. This will often prevent further losses.

PREVENTION   This is dependent on observing the precautions described earlier in the care of the syringe, avoidance of infecting the contents of the bottle, and in the technique of the inoculation.

Virus and Rickettsial Diseases

FOOT-AND-MOUTH DISEASE

Foot-and-mouth disease is a very serious and highly infectious febrile malady affecting cloven-hooved animals—cattle, swine, sheep and goats. It is characterised by severe general disturbance of health and by the local development of vesicles (small blisters or bladders) principally in the feet and in the mouth.

CAUSE   The cause is a filterable virus.

CONDITIONS OF OCCURRENCE   Although sheep are highly susceptible, when an outbreak of the disease occurs on a farm it usually first appears in the cattle or pigs.

SYMPTOMS   The incubation period varies from 48 hours to 11 days, with an average of about three or four days.

The earliest symptoms are those of dullness and loss of appetite, invariably accompanied by high fever; this stage is quickly followed by, and is often coincident with, the appearance of very severe lameness and the development of the lesions in the feet and mouth.

The lameness is usually very pronounced and is often so severe that the sheep is unable to walk, and when recumbent, may even be unable to rise. Because of this and the inability to feed and ruminate, and also because of the pain and general malaise, loss of bodily condition is very rapid; nursing mothers quickly lose their milk and pregnant ewes very often abort. When lambs are present the death-rate amongst them is heavy: in adults the condition may be rather mild.

The mouth lesions are much less common in sheep than in cattle; when present, they are neither so obvious, nor so extensive, and there may be no signs of local irritation, *eg* the profuse slavering which is invariably present in cattle. The vesicles are situated more commonly under, than upon, the lining membrane of the lips, tongue, gums or cheeks. They are very small and their presence is often difficult to determine and indeed may only become apparent when the site of the lesion is rubbed by the finger; then the overlying membrane is removed, leaving an obvious raw sore. The amount of fluid contained in the vesicle is small.

The foot lesions are more extensive and usually two or more feet are simultaneously affected. The vesicles may not be larger than a millet seed and are sometimes difficult to discover; they tend to run together and are commonly present on the heels in the skin at about its junction with the horny hoof-heads and also in the cleft between the hooves. These vesicles soon rupture, exposing raw, red sores. Because of the small size of the foot of the sheep compared with that of cattle extensive involvement of the foot may result, causing partial separation of the horny wall, which always begins from above downwards; also, as distinct from foot-rot, the horn itself is not diseased and there is a remarkable absence of proud flesh and also of suppuration—unless gross septic infection sets in. The symptoms are not, however, always very specific and diagnosis may present difficulty even to an expert.

DIAGNOSIS As has been stated it is only on rare occasions that the disease primarily attacks sheep; cattle or swine are usually the animals to be first affected. When the presence of the disease is established on a farm its eradication is in the hands of the veterinary staff of the Ministry of Agriculture, foot-and-mouth disease being notifiable under the Diseases of Animals Acts.

The precise diagnosis of foot-and-mouth disease by the flockmaster should not be attempted. Any suspicion of an outbreak must at once be reported to the nearest police officer who will transmit the information to the appropriate veterinary authority. It is important to realise that *any* outbreak of lameness with involvement of the feet should be regarded with suspicion and not immediately assumed to be foot-rot or scad, particularly if several animals are affected simultaneously. When foot-and-mouth disease occurs in a flock already affected with foot-rot it may be missed, so for this reason the importance of investigating any unusual signs must be emphasised.

LOUPING-ILL

Louping-ill, or 'trembling', has been recognised for the last 150 years as the cause of serious losses in sheep stock.

CAUSE The cause of louping-ill is a virus which is transmitted from sheep to sheep through the medium of the tick, *Ixodes ricinus;* this tick in its larval or nymphal stage acquires the virus by sucking blood from an infected sheep and then transmitting it to a healthy sheep when it bites in its subsequent nymphal or adult stage respectively. Most ticks are also infected with tick-borne fever and it is thought that the double infection can increase the severity of louping-ill symptoms by increasing the chances of virus attacking the nervous system in sheep which are not 'acclimatised', *ie* immune to these diseases.

CONDITIONS OF OCCURRENCE The disease in its occurrence was at one time thought to be peculiar to Scotland and the northern part of England, extending as far south as the Yorkshire-Lancashire Border. The disease also occurs, however, in North Wales and in parts of Ireland. In Scotland it is prevalent throughout the Western and Central Highlands and in the Southern Uplands from South Ayrshire to the Tweed.

It was early recognised that louping-ill occurred only on land which was infested with the sheep-tick, and this, in conjunction with the fact that its seasonal incidence bore relationship to the periods of maximum tick activity—April, May, early June, and again in September in the west—led to the assumption that the tick transmitted the disease.

The farm animals most susceptible to the natural disease are sheep and cattle; swine and also horses are occasionally the subjects of attack.

Wild creatures such as grouse, voles and deer also carry the virus and there can be a natural circulation between them and ticks. It should be remembered, therefore, that ground which has been free of sheep for some years will still have ticks capable of passing on the disease to farm stock. Humans are also susceptible to louping-ill infection.

SYMPTOMS In sheep exposed to natural infection, symptoms occur within 6–18 days of the attachment of the ticks. The early stage of the disease—the viraemic phase—is characterised by dullness and fever which may not be noticed. This type of illness is probably the whole course of the disease in the greater number of sheep infected. In a proportion of the animals, however, the virus attacks the brain and the well-known signs of excitability, tremors—especially of the head—muscular spasms and irregularities of gait develop. Balance may be affected and the sheep be unable to stand. Later, a paralysis of one or more legs or of the hindquarters may develop. The nervous signs differ markedly in each individual.

In some outbreaks the disease is so acute that the animals are simply found dead or recumbent, able only to make paddling movements with their legs. These explosive outbreaks have mainly been described on the west coast where lambs and adult sheep of all ages have been affected.

In the young lamb the symptoms are those of marked dullness, loss of appetite and a propensity to wander, or at least to cease following the ewe. Death frequently occurs in lambs so affected within a few days, without nervous signs or diagnostic symptoms developing.

POST-MORTEM FINDINGS No gross characteristic changes can be observed at the post-mortem examination of an affected carcase, though microscopic examination of the brain shows it to have been affected.

DIAGNOSIS The symptoms of several different disease conditions, including lambing sickness and tetany, bear considerable resemblance to those of louping-ill and there is often great difficulty in reaching even a provisional diagnosis of the disease in an individual case in the field; lambing sickness and tetany, however, affect only ewes in late pregnancy and during lactation. The occurrence of a number of deaths in sheep which have recently been moved on to tick-infested pastures from 'clean' land should cause one to suspect louping-ill. Diagnosis, however, can be very precisely determined by laboratory examination and tests. The head and a considerable portion of the neck of a suspected case should be forwarded to a veterinary laboratory without delay. The laboratory must have the specimen within an hour or two of death to give a quick diagnosis. Blood samples from animals which have been affected for a few days are also useful.

CONTROL No specific curative treatment is known but animals which suffer severe damage to the brain may recover after a fairly prolonged illness if they are carefully nursed, fed and watered. Only in rare cases, however, is such treatment attempted.

The main control of the disease results from the maintenance of a flock immunity and this, in turn, is dependent on repeated exposure to the virus.

Though an attack of the disease gives an immunity of long duration, unless this is regularly boosted the level of protective bodies in the blood falls very low. There is then little or no protection passed to the lamb in the colostrum and the lambs are often the first age group to show that the flock immunity is low, though the mothers remain apparently healthy. The typical disease is, however, most commonly diagnosed in hoggs. When, as a result of high immunity in the flock, the numbers of infected ticks on the pasture fall, lambs may never encounter the disease till they return from wintering. At this stage the death-rate can be quite appreciable. It is obvious, therefore, that there will be a fluctuation over a period of several years in the incidence of the disease and one can expect years without losses, even in the absence of vaccine. Exceptions to this are areas of very light tick infestation, or where only a part of the grazing is infested. In such circumstances losses can be unpredictable and may be very high if for some reason sheep are concentrated on the infected part at the critical time. Care must always be taken in moving sheep from infected areas when ticks are attached, as this can infect fresh ground, and even lowground pasture. Admittedly in this latter case the ticks will die out in two to three years, but in the meantime they can cause heavy loss in any sheep grazing such pasture (*see* Tick-Borne fever, page 54).

Losses from this disease could be readily controlled by an effective vaccine, but many of the worst outbreaks occur when the disease is first introduced and on infected farms heavy losses are only likely to occur on occasional years.

SCRAPIE

The disease of sheep known as 'scrapie' is a nervous disorder, characterised by symptoms of intense and progressive itch, progressive debility, and incoordination of movement.

CAUSE It has been generally accepted that the causal factor is a filterable virus located in the brain, the spinal cord, and the spleen. The disease certainly can be transmitted through the medium of the pasture, from the dam, and by inoculation, but the true nature of the cause still awaits precise determination. The incubation period may be very prolonged; it appears to extend from about 18 months to two years, or even longer.

CONDITIONS OF OCCURRENCE In this country sheep are the only animals known to be affected, though goats are susceptible by contact and the disease can be naturally transmitted by inoculation and by contact from infected to healthy sheep, goats and mice.

Scrapie is very seldom observed in sheep under 18 months of age, but there appears to be no maximum to the age incidence, and cases of the disease in 9-year-old sheep of both sexes have been recorded. The most common age is $2\frac{1}{2}$–4 years old.

As has been indicated scrapie can be transmitted through the medium of the ewe, but the infective parent may itself appear perfectly healthy at the time of mating, and may never, or perhaps only after the lapse of several years, manifest the disease, although its progeny may exhibit the characteristic symptoms of scrapie at any period from 18 months of age onwards.

SYMPTOMS The onset of the disease is insidious and only an experienced shepherd may be able to recognise the earliest signs. The sheep is nervous, apprehensive, and more excitable than usual. If closely watched, fine tremors are observed extending over the head and neck and causing slight but very rapid nodding movements. If the animal is rounded up it becomes tense with excitement and fine muscular tremors, particularly affecting the thighs and flanks, are evident. The head and neck are carried high and somewhat stiffly, the facial expression is staring and fixed, the ears not infrequently assume an unnatural position, and grinding movements of the teeth and thirst are frequent symptoms. There is no diarrhoea, but if the animal becomes excited, quantities of faeces and urine may be involuntarily passed at short intervals. The fleece becomes lighter in colour and loses its lustre. The bleating is somewhat feeble, husky, and tremulous.

The most characteristic clinical feature is the development of itch which frequently commences in the region of the rump and loins and gradually extends over the whole body. When the skin, particularly that of the back, is rubbed, the 'scratch reflex'—nibbling movements of the lips and vigorous wagging of the tail—is shown; in many instances the itch becomes extreme and the animal is unable to rest for any length of time.

Although the appetite remains unaffected almost throughout the entire course, feeding and rumination may be imperfectly performed because of the severe skin irritation. The sheep repeatedly rubs itself against fixed objects but, apart from the abrasions on the skin and the loss of wool which consequently result, no lesion of the skin is observable. As a result probably of the constant torment of irritation, emaciation and weakness are progressive in some cases and inability to rise is a common feature of the later stages, though this is often due to the characteristic motor nervous disturbances which include staggering, convulsions and paralysis of the hindquarters. Indeed, in some cases the inco-ordination may be the only sign noticed.

When scrapie attacks a nursing ewe the lamb usually remains in perfect health so long as it receives a sufficiency of milk. While itch is a characteristic feature of the disease it may be comparatively mild in degree, and in rare instances no appreciable skin irritation is evident. The symptoms tend to increase in intensity throughout the course of the disease. Scrapie is generally regarded as invariably fatal, although upon relatively rare occasions there have been cases in which spontaneous and complete recovery apparently took place.

The course of the disease shows marked variation in its duration. Instances are known in which death occurred within 14 days after the first observable signs of illness, but usually the malady is chronic in type and runs a course of six weeks to six months, or even longer, before terminating in death.

When the disease is established in a flock the incidence presents wide variation and commonly falls between 4 per cent and 20 per cent. In some flocks the incidence is so low that only occasional cases occur in a period of several years.

Post-mortem Findings   In diseases that run a chronic course it is to be expected that definite gross tissue damage will result. In this respect scrapie presents a singular exception to the general rule because, while the course is usually protracted and the symptoms become progressively more intense until death occurs, apart from the emaciation and the presence of such injuries as may have been induced by the vigorous rubbing of the skin, no gross pathological change occurs in the disease.

Diagnosis   Scrapie is to be differentiated from parasitic skin diseases, lice, etc. Usually in parasitic infestation several members of the flock show various degrees of skin irritation at about the same time; on the other hand, scrapie usually appears in single members of the flock, and then only at irregular intervals. In scrapie there is an absence of skin lesions other than those occasioned by rubbing against fixed objects. Sheep scab also causes severe itch, but this disease has been eliminated from this country.

Scrapie can be diagnosed in the laboratory by microscopic examination of certain parts of the brain.

Prevention   No specific curative or preventive treatment is known. The affected sheep should at once be removed from the pasture. Culling the offspring of affected ewes will help, and where the incidence is high this necessitates the tagging of all ewes and lambs. No affected ewe should be retained so that she may nurse her lamb as this will have the effect of spreading the infection.

CONTAGIOUS PUSTULAR DERMATITIS (Orf)

Contagious pustular dermatitis or, as it is more generally known, 'orf', is a specific contagious disease of the skin of sheep and goats, characterised by the development of proliferative scabby lesions on the lips, nose, coronet and, occasionally, the genital regions.

Cause   The cause is a filterable virus of the pox group of viruses.

Conditions of Occurrence   This disease tends to show a marked seasonal incidence, the two most common peaks being just after lambing and in the late summer. In the former case the disease appears on the mouths of the lambs and the udders of the ewes, while in the latter the feet are most commonly affected, with occasional lesions on the lips and nose. Outbreaks of the facial type can, however, occur at any time throughout the summer. Sheep of all ages are susceptible and lambs and hoggs may be attacked outwith the usual time. Older animals may be affected in the genital regions at mating time.

Symptoms   Usually the first signs seen are the appearance of scabs on the affected areas. If other members of the flock are then examined little pustules may be found at the corners of the lips and on the skin of the fetlock where it joins the hoof. These pustules run together and rupture to form the brownish scab which is usually the first noticeable sign. The scab rapidly thickens to form a prominent lesion which may vary from the size of a shilling to involvement of the whole muzzle or coronet. The incubation period from infection to visible lesion is four to five days. If the crust is removed the underlying tissues are red, moist and painful and the scab rapidly forms again on the lips. The coronet lesion tends to be red and bulging with variable amounts of scab.

In the sucking lamb the disease assumes its most severe form, though occasionally outbreaks are noticeably mild in nature. The lips are thickened and armour-plated with the hard scab which makes sucking difficult. Lesions appear on the teats of the ewe through contact with the concentrated infection of the lesions on the lamb, and though these lesions on the ewe are rarely serious in themselves, their position on the teats renders them so because mastitis, which at best destroys the affected udder and at worst may lead to the death of the ewe, is a not infrequent sequel. The pain of the lesion results in the ewe refusing the lamb which then tries in desperation to steal milk, with consequent spread of the disease. The most distressing aspect of this disease in its severe form is the accumulation of starving lambs. The death-rate in such lambs can be heavy.

In older lambs the consequences are usually less severe, but the condition persists in the flock for many weeks as fresh cases develop and the affected animals may suffer a more or less severe check.

In July, August and September the form commonly seen occurs as a prominent lesion on the coronet and occasionally further up the leg. Strawberry-like lesions may appear on the lips, probably as a result of nibbling or rubbing the foot lesions. The lesions usually affect one or two feet only, but occasionally all four feet are affected. They heal in 10–20 days but on occasion they become rather like large soft warts in character and persist, especially on the lips, for some weeks; such lesions form prominent red bulging sores, usually about the size of half a crown.

Genital orf is rather uncommon and occurs in flocks which usually have no history of orf infection. It always appears at tupping time and results in poor conception rates and long drawn out lambing. Lesions are generally confined to the prepuce of the ram and the vulva of the ewe.

Orf is rarely fatal, except in very young lambs. In occasional very severe outbreaks, however, infection may spread to the inside of the mouth and as a result of secondary infection lambs may die from toxaemia and pneumonia.

DIAGNOSIS The disease has been confused with foot-and-mouth disease and if there is any doubt, veterinary opinion must be sought immediately. If foot-and-mouth disease is suspected, the condition must immediately be reported to the police. Orf can be confirmed in the laboratory by transmission to susceptible sheep.

TREATMENT AND PREVENTION This is rarely practical because of the numbers involved and little can be done except to control the secondary invaders with antibiotics. Aerosol sprays are particularly useful for this purpose.

When disease does break out in the lambing flock, immediate removal of affected lambs and their mothers will limit the spread of the disease. If only one field is affected great care should be taken not to transfer infection to other fields on hands and clothing or, more important, by actual contact with affected lambs. Vaccines are available and when used at the correct time give reasonable protection. The vaccine is, however, made from living virus and should only be used with considerable care, especially in flocks where the disease has not previously occurred, as vaccination could be the means of introducing the disease to the farm. For this reason it is unwise to mix vaccinated with unvaccinated stock for three to four weeks after inoculation. On the Scottish Borders hoggs are usually vaccinated in June or early July, the vaccine being applied to scarification inside the thigh. Where in-lamb ewes have to be vaccinated, this should be done behind the elbow to keep infection away from the udder.

ULCERATIVE DERMATOSIS

There is some doubt as to the existence of this condition in Scotland, but outbreaks have been seen which suggest that it may be present. The form in which it is most commonly recognised is that which affects sheep in the breeding season with ulcerative lesions on the vulva of the ewe and the prepuce of the ram. It is also reported as causing an orf-like lesion around the mouth of the ewe.

The lesion differs from orf in that it is an ulcer rather than the 'strawberry-like' lesion of orf. The lesions, both on the genitalia and on the face, may become infected with bacteria, producing a purulent sore. The disease is spread by direct contact, hence its importance at mating, which it can markedly affect if it appears early in the season.

DIAGNOSIS This requires a laboratory examination using sheep susceptible to orf and immune sheep to show the presence of a different virus. There is no vaccine against this condition, which tends to affect older sheep.

TREATMENT Palliative treatment with antibiotic aerosols helps to keep down secondary infection but has little effect on the virus. Lesions on the mouth, legs and face may take three weeks to two months to heal.

PREVENTION At the first sign of the disease, especially at mating, all infected animals should be drawn out and the rams removed from the flock. After ten days an examination should reveal any further cases. Clean rams may then be put with the clean flock.

PERIORBITAL ECZEMA (Eye Scab)

This disease commonly appears just before lambing time. The lesion begins as a red, swollen area, usually just above the eye. This rapidly spreads and a black scab forms round the eye which may be completely closed. Other lesions may appear on the nose. The lesions bleed readily and badly affected sheep present an alarming appearance.

CAUSE The disease is undoubtedly contagious and spreads when the animals are at the boxes feeding. While orf virus has been isolated on occasion, it is doubtful if it is the cause in all cases and ulcerative dermatosis virus may be involved. On occasion infection spreads to the eye with loss of sight, but generally recovery is uneventful. The disease does not usually spread to the lambs.

SHEEP PULMONARY ADENOMATOSIS (Jaagsiekte)

Sheep pulmonary adenomatosis is a disease of importance but may be overlooked when individual cases occur, it being diagnosed as pneumonia. On occasion, however, losses can be rather heavy.

CAUSE The cause has not yet been determined; a filterable virus is suspected.

CONDITIONS OF OCCURRENCE The disease usually affects sheep that are more than one year old. There is good evidence that the disease can be spread by contact, indeed the origin of most outbreaks can usually be traced to one particular group of sheep brought on to the farm. The incubation period is prolonged and several months elapse between exposure to infection and the appearance of symptoms.

The first signs of the disease can be observed at any time of year. One or more sheep may show signs of troubled breathing and shortness of breath. Although the condition may be slow to develop it is invariably fatal. The next year an increasing number of animals may show these symptoms. Thereafter, the disease tends to persist in the flock. At certain periods its presence may be obvious. These periods may alternate with others of relatively long duration when the flockmaster might quite wrongly suppose that the disease had disappeared.

SYMPTOMS The disease is insidious and runs a chronic course, and even in advanced cases it is often difficult to observe symptoms of obvious illness in affected individuals other than the 'lift' seen in pneumonia. The symptoms are more readily observed after sheep have been driven or gathered from the hill. Then an affected sheep may be likely to show difficulty in respiration accompanied by an occasional soft, spasmodic cough and a thin, clear or frothy nasal discharge which may be very profuse. If one listens carefully to the chest wall of affected sheep soft, bubbling sounds, which have been aptly likened to those produced by 'slowly boiling porridge', may be heard. If the hind limbs are raised, clear fluid may run from the nostrils.

Affected sheep may die within a week or two, but generally the disease progresses much more slowly and may persist for six months or even a year before death finally occurs. During this time the appetite is maintained, although in the later stages weakness and emaciation become very evident. The disease is often complicated by a terminal bacterial pneumonia.

POST-MORTEM FINDINGS The lungs are enlarged and more or less extensively solidified. In colour they are greyish-white, mottled with purple areas. When the greyish areas are cut open they are found to consist of numerous small nodules which do not protrude above the cut surface.

DIAGNOSIS A definite diagnosis can be made only by microscopic examination of preparations of lung tissue.

CONTROL   There is no known specific method of cure or prevention. When the presence of the disease is discovered the whole flock should be carefully examined by a veterinarian and suspected cases ruthlessly culled and slaughtered. This examination should be repeated whenever practicable for a period of at least one year.

Sheep that are known to be affected should not be sold in the open market because in this way the disease can be introduced into a healthy flock.

TICK-BORNE FEVER

CAUSE   The cause of tick-borne fever is a minute, microscopic parasite, (a 'Rickettsia-like body') which can be demonstrated in certain of the white blood cells. As in louping-ill, the disease is transmitted by the bites of infected nymphal and adult ticks. The blood of infected sheep remains infective for prolonged periods; consequently, the great majority of ticks on infected pastures are likely to harbour the causal microbe, and thus where the tick infestation is heavy, probably every sheep on such pastures becomes infected by the disease.

CONDITIONS OF OCCURRENCE   Since the tick is the transmitting agent common to both diseases, tick-borne fever has the same geographical distribution and the same periods of seasonal occurrence as louping-ill. Tick-borne fever, however, has a higher incidence than louping-ill and is nearly always present on tick-infested ground, whether infected with louping-ill or not.

The great majority of lambs on pasture heavily infested with tick become infected with tick-borne fever shortly after birth. The disease in lambs is usually so mild in character that its presence is not recognised; however, it may predispose the affected animals to other diseases, of which the most important are louping-ill and tick pyaemia.

An attack of tick-borne fever renders an animal more or less immune to, or at least tolerant of, further attacks and this tolerance is reinforced at each season of tick activity so that serious manifestations of tick-borne fever are rarely seen in home-bred stock. This repeated exposure to the disease gives the animal its high degree of immunity and for this reason home-bred stock possess an 'acclimatisation value'. If, however, sheep from tick-free pastures are brought on to tick-infested areas, more severe attacks of tick-borne fever may occur, often resulting in serious losses. Cases have also been reported of high mortality in sheep returned to tick pastures after away-wintering; clinical cases also occur in a flock where the pastures are very lightly infested with tick, presumably because of waning resistance or even because these sheep escape infestation early in life, especially where only part of the hill is tick-infested. When tick-infested sheep have been brought on to tick-free pastures there have been instances of severe outbreaks of tick-borne fever in susceptible sheep grazing these pastures the following year.

SYMPTOMS   After an incubation period of about one week, symptoms of dullness develop, accompanied by a high fever and a considerable loss of physical condition. The febrile symptoms are irregular and may be prolonged, but usually subside after a period of ten days. Susceptible ewes which become infected and develop febrile symptoms during late pregnancy commonly abort (kebbing).

Attacks of the disease in susceptible sheep reduce bodily condition and general health and, as has been indicated, render the sheep more susceptible to other diseases such as pyaemia, joint-ill, louping-ill and pneumonia. Such sheep may take many weeks to recover from an attack.

POST-MORTEM FINDINGS   No specific changes at post-mortem are recognised, although enlargement of the spleen may be observed.

DIAGNOSIS   A precise diagnosis can be obtained only by laboratory tests; these consist of demonstrating the parasite in the white blood cells and of reproducing the disease in experimental sheep by inoculating blood from the suspected case.

PREVENTION   No satisfactory method of prevention by means of vaccines or sera has yet been evolved. Early exposure of sheep to the tick reduces the ill effects. Pregnant animals which come from tick-free areas must never be exposed.

CONTAGIOUS OPHTHALMIA (Heather Blindness)

Contagious ophthalmia is a specific disease of sheep that is common to most sheep-raising countries, including Scotland, where it is often referred to as 'heather blindness'.

CAUSE   A micro-organism named *Rickettsia conjunctivae* is said to be the causal agent of this disease.

CONDITIONS OF OCCURRENCE   Lambs and sheep under one year old are more commonly attacked, but sheep of all ages are susceptible. Although recovered cases develop considerable resistance to reinfection, they often remain carriers of the infection for several months and recurrences of the disease in affected flocks may appear annually, especially if fresh stock is introduced. When the disease occurs in a uniform lot of young sheep, as in recently-weaned lambs on close grazing, the spread of the infection is usually rapid and the incidence of cases may frequently be very high. It is believed that the disease is spread by the transmission to healthy sheep of droplets discharged from the eyes of affected animals.

SYMPTOMS   Infection results primarily in conjunctivitis (inflammation of the membrane lining the eyelids and the surface of the eyeball). There is at this time an excessive watery discharge from the eyes which are tender and sensitive to light. Both eyes usually become affected but a day or two may elapse between the affection of each eye. In mild cases, the first signs of recovery may be noted a few days after the onset of symptoms. On the other hand, if the attack is severe, a part or the whole of the surface of the eyeball may become cloudy and opaque, the watery discharge becomes thick, even pus-like, and temporary blindness results.

Ulceration of the eyeball may occur in some cases, and although blindness may persist in severely affected animals for three or four weeks or even longer, eventual recovery without apparent permanent damage to the eye structures almost invariably follows. The disease can be dangerous in ewes in late pregnancy since twin lamb disease (pregnancy toxaemia) can result from the severe check the animal receives. Ewes which are severely affected should be kept separate from the others and their full ration should be ensured.

DIAGNOSIS Contagious ophthalmia should at once be suspected if more than one sheep shows symptoms at about the same time.

TREATMENT Care should be taken to ensure that blind animals are prevented from injuring themselves and that they receive adequate food and water. Certain antibiotics applied as eye ointments are of definite curative value, although in the great majority of cases recovery takes place spontaneously. It appears, however, that while the antibiotic is curative while being used, the condition tends to recur when treatment is stopped. The use of these preparations is therefore usually restricted to the worst cases. The tetracyclines are reported to give best results.

ENTROPION

This condition is the result of an inturned lower eyelid which brings the eyelashes against the eyeball. The condition is included here, though it is not of an infective nature, because it is so frequently confused with ophthalmia.

The condition affects very young lambs and is usually considered hereditary. There seems little doubt that conformation at least plays a part, but there is some evidence that cold dry winds exacerbate the condition. The importance of the disease lies in the fact that, if neglected, it can result in blindness following on ulceration.

TREATMENT Mild cases may respond to manually correcting the inturned eyelid and the application of an eye ointment containing a little local anaesthetic, but most cases require surgery. Simpler methods which do not involve an incision are claimed to be equally effective. Here the eyelid is rolled outwards to its normal position and a small fold of skin below the rim is tied or fastened with a small surgical clip to retain the eyelid in position.

Functional Disorders

PINE

The term 'pine' or 'vinquish' has been generally applied to a number of disease conditions characterised by progressive debility, which affect young sheep and cattle; such conditions include round-worm infestation, Johne's disease, malnutrition and mineral deficiencies.

CAUSE The disease discussed here is specifically one of 'trace element' deficiency, the element being cobalt.

It had been shown that 'pine', a disease of young sheep and cattle which occurred in the Inner Hebrides, was closely similar to, if not identical with, a disease in New Zealand named 'bush sickness' because, apart from other considerations, both could be prevented and cured by the administration of crude iron compounds. Later investigations proved that 'bush sickness' was, in fact, due to a deficiency of cobalt. It is now known that the beneficial effects of crude iron compounds on pine are due to the fact that they contain minute quantities of cobalt as an impurity.

The role of cobalt in promoting growth and in maintaining health in the young ruminant is still imperfectly understood, but it is known that the presence of cobalt in the paunch is necessary for the proper functioning of certain bacteria which are intimately concerned both in digestion and in protein metabolism. More important, they are necessary to other bacteria which are involved in the production of the essential vitamin B_{12}. Growth and nutrition in the young ruminant animal are seriously, even vitally, impaired if cobalt is deficient in the diet.

SYMPTOMS The symptoms of pine are observed only in ruminants and are progressive debility and emaciation. The onset is frequently insidious. The affected animal is dull and the fleece becomes dry, lustreless, and broken; the visible mucous membranes, especially those within the eyelids, are pale; the physical condition is gradually lost, the eyeball becomes sunken, and there is commonly a watery discharge from the eyes. Thereafter, the weakness and emaciation progress until finally the animal is unable to rise. In lambs, growth is markedly retarded and they soon present a stunted, unthrifty appearance. In many instances the symptoms are aggravated by a superimposed round-worm infestation, but unless the worm infestation is heavy, diarrhoea does not often occur. The death-rate may be very high; on some farms it has reached 30 per cent. Loss of appetite results in a still lower intake of cobalt, completing a vicious circle.

The symptoms described are those of the acute type of pine but the disease frequently takes a much less acute form. The gradations in the intensity of the symptoms are presumably due to the varying degrees of cobalt deficiency in different pastures. In many instances the condition could be more properly described as one of poor health rather than definite disease, *ie* animals not doing as well as they should.

Post-mortem Findings The post-mortem findings are usually those of advanced emaciation.

Diagnosis Because the symptoms of cobalt-deficiency pine, Johne's disease and round-worm infestation are in many ways similar, and since worms and pine are also frequently associated, it is often very difficult, if not impossible, to form a precise diagnosis at the first examination of the flock; but a history, over a period of years, of regular occurrence of a debilitating disease affecting a considerable number of the young, immature members of the flock is suggestive of cobalt deficiency.

The mapping-out of cobalt-deficient areas can be done only with the help of a soil chemist. In the absence of a precise diagnosis, a marked response to the administration of the mineral to pining sheep will indicate cobalt deficiency.

Treatment and Prevention Cobalt must be administered so that it reaches the rumen or paunch; injection is quite useless. It has been found that any heavy object swallowed by a sheep comes to rest in the fore-stomachs and this fact has led to the making of a cobalt 'bullet' which dissolves very slowly over a period of years to give a continual supply of the element. The tiny amount required—one ounce of a cobalt salt will supply the needs of 1,000 sheep for a week—is supplied in this way.

In some cases, particularly in suckling lambs, the bullet may become coated with a deposit of a calcium salt which renders it ineffective and because of this the bullet should not be given until the lambs are weaned. Regular dosing is, of course, effective but impractical, except perhaps for diagnostic confirmation, but to be really effective dosing twice weekly is necessary. The method usually recommended is to dissolve one ounce of cobalt sulphate in a pint of water to form the stock solution; one fluid ounce of this solution is mixed with a gallon of water for dosing, each animal being given one ounce of the diluted drench. The dose can, however, be increased where the condition is acute. The cobalt may also be introduced into the normal feed, but since this may prove uneconomic a small medicated feed once a week would be more practical. Medicated salt licks, though useful, have limitations.

Undoubtedly the most useful method, where this is at all practical, is the application of cobalt as a top-dressing to pastures. The cobalt must be mixed with artificial manures, lime or sand. In New Zealand it has been found that five ounces per acre will prevent pine for a year when applied in the autumn, but, in this country, two pounds per acre is the amount generally recommended. This is said to be effective for three years.

Cobalt deficiency may co-exist with copper deficiency and this should be considered when a deficiency of either of these elements is suspected. Certain areas are well-known to be deficient in cobalt but in others the low level of the

1 Vaccination 'abscesses'. This shoulder illustrates the effect of indiscriminate choice of vaccination site.

2 Spinal abscess. Note the characteristic 'sitting dog' posture of the lamb.

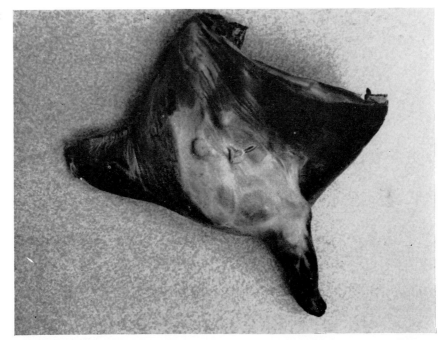

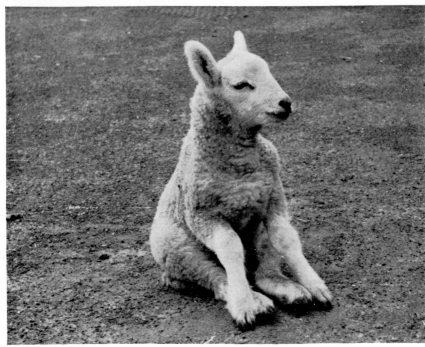

3   Mycotic dermatitis affecting the face.

4   Peri-orbital eczema. This shows the rather startling appearance of a severely affected ewe.

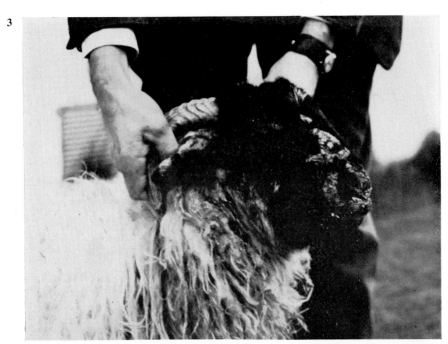

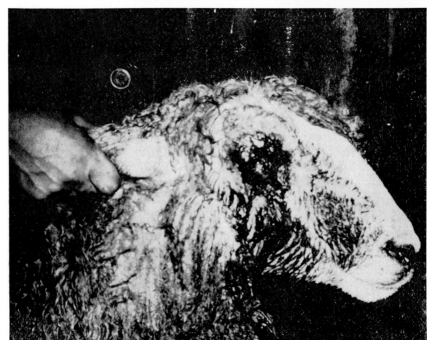

element comes to light when land is improved and fertilised. Individual fields on a farm may be affected.

SWAYBACK

Swayback is a disease of the nervous system affecting young lambs.

CAUSE Swayback is caused by faulty development of the brain and spinal cord of the lamb as a result of defective copper metabolism in the ewe. The tissues of both the ewe and the affected lamb are deficient in copper though the grazings can have this element in adequate quantity. Since the administration of copper to the pregnant ewe will prevent the disease in the lamb it would seem that for some reason the affected ewe is unable to use the copper in the herbage.

CONDITIONS OF OCCURRENCE The disease occurs at two fairly well-defined times in the life of the lamb—at birth or, in lambs which are normal at birth, at ten days to six weeks of age. There is considerable variation in the degree of severity, with the most severe cases occurring earlier. The disease is widespread but is more prevalent in certain districts where it occurs annually in varying incidence, being particularly prevalent following mild and open winters when little or no supplementary feeding is given and, also, when growth of herbage occurs in the last weeks of pregnancy. Improvement of marginal and hill pastures with liming and reseeding may cause a sharp rise in the incidence of swayback or lead to its appearance on farms where it was previously unknown. In Scotland, areas with a southerly aspect are worst affected. While the disease occurs in lambs of all breeds and crosses, some breeds, such as the Blackface, appear more susceptible than others.

SYMPTOMS In the lamb born with the condition, the signs may be rather vague. In severe cases the lamb cannot rise or support itself if lifted to its feet; in mild cases all that may be noticed is a slight irregularity of movement of the hind limbs, particularly when the lamb attempts to run. All degrees of abnormality between these two extremes may be seen.

In older lambs the signs of the disease, often called delayed swayback, are much more characteristic and are more readily diagnosed clinically. The lamb may run several steps in an apparently normal fashion, then suddenly collapse on one hip rather like a dog sitting down. This collapse is accompanied by a turning movement which may swing the lamb right round to face the opposite direction.

The duration of the disease is very variable. A new born lamb, acutely affected, may live only a few hours. Less acute cases may die from starvation, since they are unable to follow the ewe or to support themselves while sucking. Delayed swayback rarely results in death from the disease itself but, as movement becomes more and more difficult, the lamb may die from pneumonia or other intercurrent disease. Affected animals never recover, though the symptoms may be arrested, particularly in mild cases. These may live for a normal lifespan and even bear healthy lambs.

POST-MORTEM FINDINGS In most cases in new-born lambs, cavities may be seen in the white matter of the brain, but in very mild cases and in delayed swayback the damage is microscopic and an expert examination is necessary for definite diagnosis.

DIAGNOSIS The disease should be suspected in new-born 'weakly' lambs or lambs showing peculiarities of gait. Confirmation is obtained by post-mortem examination, sometimes microscopic, of the brain. In delayed swayback the signs are so characteristic that little difficulty is experienced in making an accurate diagnosis clinically. For confirmation, a specialist microscopic examination of the brain and spinal cord is often necessary.

TREATMENT Curative treatment is not effective, though dosing may appear to arrest the development of the symptoms in mild cases. Normally, no attempt at treatment is made.

PREVENTION The disease can be largely prevented by dosing pregnant ewes with copper, either by mouth or by injection with a specially formulated preparation, four to eight weeks before lambing. On farms where the incidence is high two doses may be necessary. Always seek veterinary advice before proceeding to dose since excess copper is very poisonous to sheep. When the disease appears unexpectedly amongst the early lambs it is worthwhile to dose the ewes still to lamb as this seems to reduce appreciably the incidence in the later-lambing ewes.

Copper-fortified licks are sometimes employed but have the disadvantage that there is no guarantee that all the ewes are taking sufficient copper from them. When such licks have been used, dosing or injecting copper can be hazardous because some ewes may have a very high copper level in the liver. Copper dressing of pasture is risky and is not recommended. For these reasons, individual dosing of the ewes is to be preferred.

WHITE MUSCLE DISEASE (Stiff Lamb Disease)

This disease is rarely seen in Scotland but outbreaks involving quite large numbers of lambs occasionally occur.

CAUSE The disease is apparently related to the feeding of the ewes in pregnancy but the exact factors involved have not been definitely established.

SYMPTOMS The affected lambs show a peculiar stiff gait and weakness of the limbs. Severely affected cases may be unable to stand.

POST-MORTEM FINDINGS Groups of muscles are seen to be very pale in colour, hence the name white muscle disease.

PREVENTION While present knowledge does not enable definite dietary recommendations to be made, the administration of selenium to the pregnant ewe or—where the disease has been diagnosed—to the new-born lamb will reduce the incidence. This substance should be administered only under the direction of a veterinary surgeon.

DOUBLE SCALP

The condition known as 'double scalp', 'double scaup', 'scappie' or 'cappi' is the result of a generalised defective formation of bone (osteoporosis) in which the bone which is formed is normal, but there is too little of it.

CAUSE The cause remains unknown, but evidence suggests that the condition may be due to a nutritional deficiency of protein allied to defects in mineral metabolism.

In most cases the disease is associated with a heavy burden of gastro-intestinal round worms. Although worm burdens lead to a rapid deterioration in the lambs' condition and tend to increase in any pining or debilitating condition (*see* Parasitic Gastro-Enteritis, page 94) they are not an essential factor in the cause of double scalp.

CONDITIONS OF OCCURRENCE The geographical distribution of the disease has yet to be accurately determined. It is seen mainly on the poorer hill grazings of the north of England and the south of Scotland where supplementary feeding is not normally provided; but a great deal more knowledge is still needed. Double scalp is most commonly seen in young sheep during the first autumn and winter of their lives, but it can affect sheep of any age. Its occurrence in breeding ewes is thought to be due to their having been affected as lambs and making an apparent recovery, with the disease recurring later under the strain of pregnancy and lactation.

SYMPTOMS The affected animal appears unthrifty, with a poor and lustreless fleece; the frontal bones of the skull are thin and yielding and sometimes fracture when pressure is applied to the area between the eyes. Symptoms of a worm burden are often present as well, and include scouring, anaemia, a watery discharge from the eyes and some degree of dropsical swelling in the region of the lower jaw.

The condition continues throughout the winter months when the nutritional value of hill grazings is at its lowest level. A marked improvement in the condition of affected animals usually occurs with the first flush of new grass in the spring.

POST-MORTEM FINDINGS The post-mortem appearances are those associated with anaemia and debility. The body cavities contain varying amounts of dropsical fluid; the heart muscle is pale and flabby and there is an absence of fat throughout the body.

The long bones are abnormally light and delicate in appearance and in extreme cases their density is reduced. They are no softer than normal, however, do not show distortion and have little tendency to fracture easily. The flat bones are considerably reduced in thickness and consist of very delicate and porous tissue covered by an extremely thin layer of compact bone. These changes are particularly notable in the frontal bone, in which the condition can be easily recognised during life and from which it takes its name.

DIAGNOSIS   While it is possible to reach a diagnosis on consideration of the clinical symptoms, this can be made more accurately by post-mortem examination of an affected animal.

TREATMENT   If it is at all possible the affected sheep should be removed from the hill to a sheltered grass park and provided with a supplementary ration of hay and concentrates; if this is not possible they should be moved to the most sheltered part of the hill and fed. A good mineral mixture appears to help. There is no justification for the old belief that fracturing the outer plate of the frontal bone will cure this condition!

OTHER BONE CONDITIONS

In addition to Double Scalp there are other conditions caused by nutritional deficiencies which can produce harmful effects on the bones of sheep. These are:

Rickets (Bent-Leg)

CAUSE   Lack of Vitamin D and/or a dietary deficiency of phosphorus, or an imbalance of the calcium/phosphorus ratio of the diet can cause rickets.

CONDITIONS OF OCCURRENCE   Rickets occurs only in young growing sheep, usually at about 8–12 months of age (December–April). The appearance of symptoms may be precipitated by the feeding of concentrates intended to stimulate rapid growth, where particular care has not been taken to ensure that the lamb's requirements of vitamin D and a correctly-balanced calcium/phosphorus intake are adequately met. In winter, because of lack of sunlight, the young sheep cannot produce sufficient vitamin D in its own tissues to permit normal bone growth. The disease, therefore, commonly occurs in tup lambs which are kept indoors or are fed generously during the winter. It is usually confined to the tup lambs even though the ewe lambs are being similarly treated.

SYMPTOMS   These can vary from a vague shifting lameness accompanied by unthriftiness and slight swelling of the knee, hock or pastern joints, to gross deformity with bending of the limb bones.

POST-MORTEM FINDINGS   The ends of the long bones are expanded (hence the enlargement of the joints noted in life) and on sawing them longitudinally the growth cartilages may be found to be irregularly or uniformly thickened. The junctions of the lower ends of the ribs with the sternal cartilages may also show enlargement, giving a row of bony thickenings on the chest wall—rickety rosary.

DIAGNOSIS   Where there is enlargement of the joints this presents little difficulty, but where lameness alone is apparent, chemical analysis of a blood sample to demonstrate a deficiency of phosphate becomes necessary in order to make an exact diagnosis.

TREATMENT   This consists of the administration of vitamin D, together with the provision of a concentrate supplement containing the correct proportions and amounts of calcium and phosphorus. Fed throughout the winter, this will prevent the disease. This treatment should be given under the advice of a veterinary surgeon.

Dental Mal-Occlusion (Open Mouth)

This is a form of rickets affecting the jaw-bone. It is not as common as that affecting the limb bones, but when it does occur, it may affect considerable numbers of the hoggs and can interfere seriously with their ability to graze.

CAUSE As for rickets. The dietary deficiencies cause softening of the jaw-bone which becomes deformed, probably by muscular pressure.

CONDITIONS OF OCCURRENCE Open-mouth is seen in hoggs, usually between January and April, and mostly in animals grazing poorer marginal land without supplementary feeding.

SYMPTOMS A loss of condition is the first apparent symptom. On examination it can be seen that the mouth cannot be closed and that there is a gap of from one quarter of an inch to as much as one and a half ins between the incisor teeth and the dental pad which cannot be reduced even by applying pressure to the upper and lower jaws. The lower lips may be wet because of dribbling of saliva.

DIAGNOSIS Once the symptoms are recognised diagnosis presents no problem.

TREATMENT As for rickets. Complete recovery can take place.

Osteomalacia (Cruban)

This is a condition comparable to rickets, occurring in the adult sheep. Since the limb bones have achieved their full length, the pathological changes and symptoms are somewhat different.

CAUSE As for rickets, although since it occurs in summer, lack of vitamin D may be of less importance than a deficient or imbalanced calcium-phosphorus intake.

CONDITIONS OF OCCURRENCE This disease occurs in June, July and August in hill ewes which are nursing good lambs (ewes without lambs and those rearing poorer lambs are unaffected). The herbage on hill farms is commonly deficient in calcium and phosphorus, and the most important factor in precipitating this disease is the drain on the ewe's mineral reserves brought about by heavy lactation. The highest incidence of this condition is said to occur in hot, dry summers.

SYMPTOMS A progressive stiffness with loss of condition is the first visible symptom. At first the affected ewe finds it easier to move uphill than down, but later is unwilling to move at all and tends to keep the hind limbs well in below the body. For this reason cases are commonly found on the hilltops. If clipped on the hill or, preferably, brought down to lowground, they can recover within two weeks. This condition affects ewes of three years old and upwards, gimmers only occasionally; from 10–20 per cent of the ewe flock can show symptoms.

DIAGNOSIS The clinical symptoms are usually sufficiently characteristic to enable a diagnosis to be made without any great difficulty, but confirmation depends on the demonstration of a deficiency of phosphate in the blood by chemical analysis.

TREATMENT Similar to that advised for rickets. Affected ewes should be brought down to low ground as soon as possible. The administration of vitamin D, together with the provision of a concentrate supplement containing the correct proportions and amounts of calcium and phosphorus, should be carried out under the advice of a veterinary surgeon.

PREGNANCY TOXAEMIA (Twin Lamb Disease)

Pregnancy toxaemia is a disease affecting ewes in the last few weeks of pregnancy and is usually seen in animals carrying more than one lamb. Cases in ewes carrying a single lamb are rare.

CAUSE This is now known to be rather complex but the disease is basically the result of the ewe's being unable to utilise her food properly, either because she is not being fed enough food of the right quality, or because of a metabolic upset. Thus, anything which interferes with the ewe's food intake during the last month of pregnancy can result in an outbreak, *eg* heather blindness, foot-rot, snowfall, etc, or several hours' starvation through movement of the flock, etc.

It seems likely that on occasion lowground ewes may not eat enough in late pregnancy to keep their own and the lambs' blood sugar at a sufficiently high level for health, with the result that all the sugar stored in the liver is used up. The ewe is not then able to use her stored body fat properly and disease develops. Lack of appetite in over-fat ewes is probably the reason for their developing the disease. This condition is essentially one affecting ewes on low ground. Hill ewes seldom show the recognised signs of the disease, though the symptoms of starvation are similar.

CONDITIONS OF OCCURRENCE Intercurrent disease and sudden storms have already been mentioned as simple obvious causes, but the causation can be much more complex, the disease occurring in both fat ewes and over-thin ewes for very different reasons. In the thin ewes the disease results from insufficient feeding—not necessarily in quantity but rather in quality. An example of this is when poorer silage is fed in late pregnancy or where fibre makes up most of the ration. Similarly, when trough space is inadequate, shy ewes—particularly gimmers—do not get their share of the ration. A further factor which is sometimes overlooked is the method of feeding. When ewes late in pregnancy are folded on turnips and given concentrates later, many will not eat the concentrates for an hour or two and by then the greedy feeders will have cleared the board.

SYMPTOMS These are readily confused with lambing sickness and even tetany, but in most cases the affected ewes live for three or four days compared with the few hours' duration of the other two conditions. However, the low blood calcium and magnesium connected with these two diseases may result from the ewe stopping feeding and death may occur quite quickly as a result. Affected animals are dull, cease to feed, have obvious difficulty in seeing and may be completely blind though the eye looks normal. They become uncertain in their movements, fall over and eventually cannot rise, gradually becoming more comatose till death occurs. Grinding of the teeth with a discharge from the nose are common, which together with the frequently laboured breathing, sometimes results in pneumonia being suspected. A sweet smell may often be recognised in the breath. Some ewes may abort and recovery takes place. Otherwise, in the absence of treatment, death invariably results. A number of ewes may be affected within a few days, giving the impression of an infectious disease.

DIAGNOSIS When ewes in the last month of pregnancy show these symptoms, this condition is by far the most likely. However, the similarity of the symptoms of milk fever and tetany emphasises the need for veterinary advice when they occur. Blood samples taken by the veterinary surgeon will confirm the diagnosis and also eliminate low blood calcium (lambing sickness) and low blood magnesium (tetany).

TREATMENT This is not very satisfactory unless the cases are caught in an early stage. Two to four ounces of glycerine twice a day sometimes give excellent results as does glucose injected into the vein by the vet. However, nursing is also important and this factor is often overlooked. The ewe should be moved to shelter and gently encouraged to drink. Some appetising concentrates should be placed within easy reach. The use of cortisone cannot be recommended in the present state of knowledge, though cures have been attributed to the drug. Good results are claimed when delivery of the lambs by caesarian section is carried out by a veterinary surgeon.

PREVENTION Steps to prevent the disease developing should be taken soon after tupping. The ewes at this stage should be in first class condition to encourage a high incidence of twins and three to four weeks afterwards should be put on more spartan rations with the aim of getting them in harder condition. It is important not to allow them to become too thin. This hard condition should be maintained till some eight weeks before they are due to lamb, when the aim should be to achieve a steady improvement in bodily condition till lambing. Enlargement of the abdomen due to the development of the lambs must not be confused with bodily improvement in the ewe. Any check in this progress by, for example, a storm, must be compensated by an increased ration. When turnips are being fed on the break, the concentrate ration should be given before the ewes are moved on. Avoid holding the ewes in the pens for vaccinations, etc, any longer than is necessary and avoid any unnecessary changes; when these must be made they should be done gradually.

LAMBING SICKNESS (Milk Fever)

Lambing sickness is an acute functional disease characterised by nervous symptoms affecting the pregnant and the lactating ewe and associated with a marked fall in the calcium level in the blood.

CAUSE Milk fever in the cow is due to an acute fall in the concentration of blood calcium, and the injection of assimilable calcium salts effects a rapid and complete recovery from this disease. The condition known as lambing sickness in the ewe has been shown to be closely allied to milk fever in the cow.

CONDITIONS OF OCCURRENCE Lambing sickness not infrequently appears shortly before lambing, especially if the ewe is subjected to undue exertion and fatigue such as may be occasioned by overdriving, rail or road transport, etc; it also commonly affects ewes with young lambs at foot and hill ewes brought in-bye to lamb.

SYMPTOMS In the primary phase of the attack the symptoms are spasms of certain muscles of the trunk and legs accompanied by considerable excitement and general distress; these symptoms may, however, be slight and transient and are usually very quickly followed by the comatose phase, in which the ewe lies completely prostrate and insensible. Death may result within 24 hours. If the ewe is unattended and acute distention of the abdomen develops during the coma, asphyxiation may be the immediate cause of death.

POST-MORTEM FINDINGS Very often, on post-mortem examination no lesion is recorded.

DIAGNOSIS Lambing sickness, in its clinical symptoms, bears some resemblance to pregnancy toxaemia and tetany, and it is only in recent years that the first two conditions have been clearly distinguished on clinical and pathological grounds.

Pregnancy toxaemia does not occur after lambing. When lambing sickness occurs in the pregnant ewe the disease is almost invariably associated with over-exertion and fatigue. Not infrequently, lambing sickness has been mistaken for louping-ill. Tetany is, however, the disease most likely to be confused with it and indeed the two diseases may be present in the same animal. The quick response to calcium in lambing sickness will distinguish the two conditions.

TREATMENT In this condition an immediate and spectacular response is obtained from an injection of calcium borogluconate beneath the skin. At lambing time the shepherd should carry a bottle of this preparation with him at all times, together with a sterile syringe and needles. The dose depends on the preparation used and the instructions on the bottle should be followed. It is very important that at each treatment a sterile needle be used to withdraw the fluid from the bottle as the preparation is easily contaminated. The syringe must be rinsed at once after use, in cold water. On the hill a rinse in *clean* burn water is usually sufficient, provided it is followed by a further rinse in methylated spirit.

PREVENTION There is no recognised method of preventing the disease but too violent change and forced exercise should be avoided immediately before and after lambing.

MAGNESIUM DEFICIENCY—HYPOMAGNESAEMIA (Tetany)

This disease which is allied to hypomagnesaemia in cattle ('lactation tetany') has greatly increased in incidence during recent years, or is more frequently recognised.

CAUSE   It is recognised that the immediate cause of the attack is an acute deficiency of magnesium in the blood, but the fundamental causes underlying this deficiency are not clearly understood.

CONDITIONS OF OCCURRENCE   Ewes of all breeds and of all ages may be affected but cast hill ewes transferred to enclosed lowland pastures for crossing with a mutton-type ram seem to be relatively susceptible; also ewes with twin lambs are commonly attacked.

The disease usually occurs from about a fortnight before, until about a month after, lambing. Certain pastures—particularly recently sown leys—predispose to the occurrence of the disease. The incidence of the disease is influenced by the potassium levels of the pasture and care is necessary in applying this element; the disease is most prevalent on improved marginal pasture. Cases have been shown to occur after a few hours' starvation of the ewes.

SYMPTOMS   In some instances the course of the disease may be so acute and short that the affected ewe is found dead within a few hours of a routine inspection at which she appeared to be perfectly well; indeed a sequence of sudden, unexpected deaths in the ewe flock may be the first indication of the presence of the disease. In such cases, on closer examination, several ewes may be observed to be more easily excited than usual and some may show convulsive spasms, especially when unduly agitated. During the short course of observable illness the main symptoms are those of acute convulsive seizures which usually recur in quick succession. Ewes in the early stages show a fine tremor of the facial muscles and an inability to move.

POST-MORTEM FINDINGS   The kidneys are pale with blood splashing and there is frequently blood-stained fluid round the heart. Decomposition is usually rapid.

DIAGNOSIS   This disease has been frequently confused with lambing sickness from which it cannot readily be distinguished by the symptoms alone; indeed in many instances it is possible to differentiate between the two diseases only if affected ewes fail to respond to the injection of calcium. A definite diagnosis can be reached by a chemical analysis of the blood, but because the blood sample must be collected during life and the period of observable illness is so short, this is often impracticable. It is known, however, that during an outbreak the level of blood magnesium in the flock is generally low and a diagnosis may be made from the analysis of the blood of a small number of ewes in the affected flock, even if these ewes show no evident signs of the disease. A precise diagnosis is important because it is only upon this that rational treatment can be based.

TREATMENT If an affected animal can be treated during the short course of actual attack the symptoms may be controlled by the injection of an appropriate preparation of magnesium; but relapses are likely to occur and the treatment should be repeated daily for several days. In view of the fact that calcium is also low in tetany, combined magnesium/calcium preparations should be used.

PREVENTION The disease can be largely prevented by feeding half an ounce of calcined magnesite to the ewes each day. To be effective, the magnesite should be included in a concentrate ration. As the disease is most common in the three weeks after lambing this is the period during which the supplement should be fed.

The disease is most severe on the highly manured 'early bite' which is so often kept for newly lambed ewes. It is therefore advisable to graze these ewes on older pasture for the first three weeks. When fields require liming, magnesian limestone should be used, as this will raise the level of the magnesium in the grass—the easiest way to feed a supplement. On occasion, in an emergency, pasture may be sprayed with magnesium salts. The method and the amount can be ascertained from the agricultural advisers.

YELLOWSES

Yellowses or 'head grit' is a condition almost entirely confined to lambs and hoggs. The parts affected are the ears and face in whitefaced sheep or white areas in blackface and crosses. The damage to these areas results from a process known as photosensitisation which is caused by the skin becoming sensitive to sunlight. This results from the ingestion of certain plants or drugs which, either directly or by their effect on the liver, result in these photosensitising substances entering the circulation. These have little or no effect till the animal is exposed to sunlight when the unpigmented skin, which is not protected by wool, reacts quite violently, becoming 'water-logged' or oedematous with an exudate which hardens to form a scab. As a result of the liver damage, these signs are often accompanied by jaundice which gives the disease the name 'yellowses'.

CONDITIONS OF OCCURRENCE The disease is most common in June, July and, to a lesser extent, August and the incidence varies from year to year. It is most common on rough hill pastures, though it is sometimes seen on lowground, particularly in lambs grazing rape. Bright sunlight is not necessary for the production of the disease.

CLINICAL SIGNS These are sudden in their onset with swelling of the eyelids and lips and, more particularly, in the ears, which hang down with the weight of the fluid accumulating below the skin. Fluid oozes through the skin and forms a scab while the membranes of the eye become yellowish in colour. The affected animal is dull and rapidly loses condition. The scabs may become infected and rather severe suppurating sores result. Commonly, varying areas of the ear may wither and drop off. On occasion a number of the animals may die and others show severe loss of condition with slow recovery.

POST-MORTEM FINDINGS Apart from the external signs described, jaundice of all tissues is commonly present.

TREATMENT Animals should if possible be housed in dark cattle courts or barns for several days and in any case, especially in lowground sheep, moved from the affected pasture. Antibiotic aerosols may be useful when the sores become infected.

FACE SCAB

Outbreaks of this condition, which seem to be akin to yellowes, have been seen occasionally in south Scotland over the last few summers. The disease is characterised by the appearance of hard dry crusts or scabs on the face and ears of the affected animals which may be lambs or ewes. Incidence within a flock varies considerably. The condition cannot be transmitted to other sheep and when the scabs are removed the skin is found to be intact. The disease is sudden in its onset, all cases appearing within one or two days. Thereafter, new cases rarely occur.

The appearance of the lesions and the story of the disease appear to indicate a form of the photosensitisation mentioned under yellowses; face scab, however, differs from this disease in that the affected sheep are rarely ill unless the lips are severely involved, making feeding difficult. Also, the scabs are dry and hard and there is little tendency for the ears to slough. The cause is quite unknown and though the condition has a superficial resemblance to the facial eczema of New Zealand, the liver has not been found to be damaged as it is in the New Zealand disease.

In the absence of certain knowledge of the cause it is impossible to suggest methods of control. Treatment is necessary only when the disease interferes with feeding and then takes the form of box feeding the few animals so affected. Though the scabs are slow to fall off, they do so after three or four weeks, leaving the skin unmarked.

It is important to distinguish this disease from orf to which it also bears some resemblance. The sudden appearance of the disease in a number of animals with its failure to spread after the first day or two and the healthy skin beneath the scab all serve to separate the two conditions.

Poisoning in Sheep

Apart from poisonings such as copper, rape and kale, and occasionally sodium chlorate, poisoning is rare in sheep unless the substance is administered inadvertently in dosing for worms.

Occasional deaths from acorn poisoning have been seen in park sheep and recently there has been some evidence that bracken poisoning may be important in some areas (*see* Bright Blindness, page 77). Cases of poisoning, when they do occur, are usually seen when snow makes the animals desperate enough to eat shrubs which they would normally ignore. One of the most common evergreens involved is rhododendron but other shrubs, such as laurel, are occasionally eaten. Symptoms vary according to the species and the amount consumed; poisoning should be suspected when several sheep are unaccountably found sick, dead or dying within a few hours.

Occasionally, carbon tetrachloride used for fluke treatment can, under certain rather ill-defined conditions, act as a poison resulting in quite heavy losses.

COPPER

Sheep are peculiarly susceptible to copper poisoning and care is necessary when it is used in the flock. Poisoning from a single dose is rare and is usually the result of carelessness in dosing for swayback, or in spraying orchards, etc, and then allowing sheep access. The form most commonly seen results from the feeding of very small quantities of copper over a long period. This copper is stored in the liver and may reach very high levels which can be suddenly released. The acute attack which follows may result from a therapeutic dose of copper, from stress, or even from a change of pasture. When copper levels in the ration even slightly exceed the normal found in such concentrates as grain, the sheep tends to accumulate dangerous quantities after some months or even weeks. The heavier the concentrate feeding, of course, the greater and quicker the accumulation. When the copper is released the great excess in the blood causes the red cells to break up, making the eyes and mucus membranes a dirty brownish yellow colour, similar to acute jaundice. In the early stages the animal may appear anaemic before the jaundice-like symptoms develop. The urine is red in colour. The animal invariably dies in twelve hours to three days.

POST-MORTEM FINDINGS The whole carcase is deeply stained yellow brown and the kidneys are characteristically black. The high levels of copper in the liver persist for some time even if the source of copper has been removed and deaths may occur two or three months later, especially if the animals are under any stress.

DIAGNOSIS When the signs described above are seen in sheep, they are most likely to be the result of copper poisoning, though a somewhat similar picture results from nitrate or sodium chlorate poisoning and from kale anaemia. These latter causes are usually readily eliminated by the history.

TREATMENT There is no effective treatment for sick animals. Preventive measures lie in recognising the susceptibility of the sheep to copper and avoiding an excessive intake. For this reason it is inadvisable to feed minerals containing copper to sheep except for short periods and then, under veterinary advice. Minerals available to sheep at other times should be copper-free.

Housed sheep being fed concentrates are peculiarly susceptible to copper poisoning and levels as low as 17 parts per million in the diet have resulted in fatalities after a few months. When concentrate feeding of housed animals is practised, therefore, steps should be taken to ensure that the copper level in the ration is less than 12–14 parts per million.

When copper is used to counteract a deficiency it should be given as a measured dose or injection. If, however, copper minerals and licks have been provided, it may be dangerous to dose or inject. Keep sheep away from concentrate feeds formulated for other stock, especially pigs, for these may contain copper levels highly dangerous for sheep, though harmless and even beneficial to the stock for which they were devised.

KALE AND RAPE

(a) Jaundice

Because of climatic or other conditions (the nature of which is not yet understood) sheep that are entirely restricted to a diet of kale or rape may occasionally develop a form of jaundice. The actual agent—or agents—which these plants activate, and by so doing, become dangerous, is as yet unknown. Rarely, cases occur with sprouting turnips as the causative factor.

SYMPTOMS These are marked by signs of deep dejection; the head droops, the back is arched and the eyes are sunken. Respiration and pulse are much increased in rate. The lining membranes of the eyes and mouth are yellow-brown in colour and there is also yellowish discolouration of the skin. The urine is noticeably dark in appearance. If the animals remain on the affected feed the condition often proves fatal.

In occasional incidents nervous signs are marked and jaundice is not seen in such cases.

POST-MORTEM FINDINGS The most striking feature is the deep yellowish discolouration of all the organs in the body. It will be noticed that the liver is bright yellow-brown and that the kidneys are yellowish-black in colour. The gall bladder is usually much distended.

TREATMENT If the condition is diagnosed early enough, affected animals quickly recover when they are taken off the kale or rape.

PREVENTION Sheep should not be confined to grazings consisting only of kale or rape; an occasional change to grass is an important preventive measure.

A condition similar in its symptoms to kale poisoning may be produced by copper poisoning (*see* page 70) and by nitrate and sodium chlorate poisoning.

(*b*) **Goitre**

When pregnant ewes are continuously fed on kale both they and their newborn lambs may suffer from a form of goitre. This condition is, however, relatively rare and would appear to be quite distinct from the form of jaundice described above.

SYMPTOMS The affected ewes are somewhat 'soft' and less energetic than normal and their udders tend to be under-developed. The lambs of such ewes are weak at birth and may even be unable to stand. Several such lambs may show signs of mental abnormality and, almost invariably, death occurs within a few days.

In addition to these symptoms evidence of goitre may be observed—both in the ewe and lamb—in a marked enlargement of the thyroid gland which is situated in the upper part of the neck.

PREVENTION Ewes during pregnancy should be fed kale only in limited amounts.

RHODODENDRON

While many plants are capable of poisoning sheep it is comparatively rare for these animals to eat poisonous plants. Exceptionally, a few sheep are sometimes poisoned by cuttings from garden plants; rhododendron poisoning is the most common and occurs when snowfall is heavy and prolonged. Animals are usually found dead but may be seen salivating, kicking at their bellies and even attempting to vomit. There is no treatment likely to be helpful.

PREVENTION Care should be taken that rhododendron and other poisonous evergreens are kept out of the reach of sheep.

Miscellaneous Conditions

DAFT LAMBS (Dafties) (Inherited Cortical Cerebellar Atrophy)

'Daftness' is a congenital abnormality which occurs principally in lambs of the Border Leceister breed and its crosses; it is much less frequently observed in other breeds. The disease occurs in widely separated areas throughout Britain but the flock incidence in any one year is usually very low. 'Daft' lambs are carried to full-term and are usually in quite good physical condition at birth.

CAUSE The cause is unknown but it is almost certainly an inherited disorder.

SYMPTOMS The symptoms of the disease are obvious at, or shortly after, birth. Individual cases vary considerably in severity; some cases are unable to walk or even to stand, while others can move about at will, although with difficulty. Typically, the head is carried very high with the muzzle pointing upwards or even pulled backwards over the neck or towards one side. The neck muscles are tense and stiff. When walking is possible, progression is often in small circles; the animal may step backwards or kneel on its forelegs. The facial expression and abnormal behaviour suggest stupidity—a general blunting of the senses—hence the name 'daftness'. In all cases there is great difficulty in sucking the mother and the lamb may quickly die from starvation; less severely affected lambs will reach adult age if able to suck, or if reared artificially on the bottle. As the young animal grows older the symptoms tend to become less severe and in adult ewes they may be apparent only when the sheep is excited, *eg* at dipping time.

POST-MORTEM FINDINGS No gross abnormality can be observed but microscopic examination of the brain reveals degenerative changes in certain important nerve cells.

DIAGNOSIS The nature of the condition is suggested by the symptoms which, however, may be confused with those of swayback. Precise diagnosis is dependent on laboratory examination.

TREATMENT AND PREVENTION There is no known curative treatment and recovered cases should not be retained in the breeding flock since they may transmit the disease to their offspring. Sires known to pass on 'daftness' to their progeny should be eliminated from the flock.

RED FOOT

'Red foot' is a disease of young lambs in which the horn of the hooves becomes detached and may be shed, leaving the red, sensitive tissue exposed. This condition may be accompanied by ulcerated areas on the membrane lining the mouth cavity. Blackface lambs are the breed usually affected.

CAUSE The cause is unknown but the available evidence does not indicate that the disease is due to an infective agent.

CONDITIONS OF OCCURRENCE The disease occurs in low incidence but is widely distributed on farms in southern and central Scotland; it appears to be of very rare occurrence in the northern Scottish counties. The incidence in affected hirsels rarely exceeds 1 per cent. The condition occurs in one or more feet very shortly after birth.

SYMPTOMS Because of the detachment of the horny hoof the lamb is so crippled that it is unable to follow and suck the ewe, and in consequence quickly dies from starvation.

TREATMENT The disease process is still quite obscure and rational means of prevention are therefore not known. The incurable nature of the lesion in the very young lamb is such that treatment is out of the question. Immediate destruction is the only proper course.

BORDER DISEASE

This is a condition which is present in the lamb at birth and derives its name from the fact that it was first recognised in the Border counties between England and Wales.

CAUSE Experimentally, the disease may be transmitted by the inoculation of tissues from affected lambs into pregnant ewes, so it must be considered as a transmissible and therefore infectious disease.

CONDITIONS OF OCCURRENCE On farms where the disease has been present for some time, cases tend to be most numerous in the offspring of hoggs and gimmers. Where the condition appears for the first time the incidence may be high in lambs from older ewes also. The disease has not so far been confirmed in Scotland, though suspect cases have been encountered.

SYMPTOMS Border disease is evident from the appearance of lambs with an unusual birth-coat. Affected animals have an abnormally coarse (and sometimes pigmented) fleece for the breed concerned, with varying amounts of fine 'halo hairs' which stand out from the birth-coat proper. There is often an abnormally high death-rate in the lambs, which do not thrive. There may also be a history of abortion and unusually poor lambing percentages. A variable proportion of cases also have a nervous disorder—a characteristic coarse tremor of trunk and limbs. Such lambs are called 'shakers'. If they can be kept alive for a few months the nervous symptoms may disappear, but such lambs tend to remain ill-thriven and death may occur quite suddenly at any time.

5 Abortion. Toxoplasmosis. Typical appearance of mummified foetus.

6 Abortion. Toxoplasmosis. The cotyledons in this fresh specimen show the typical white spots.

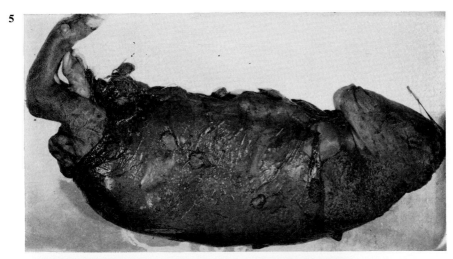

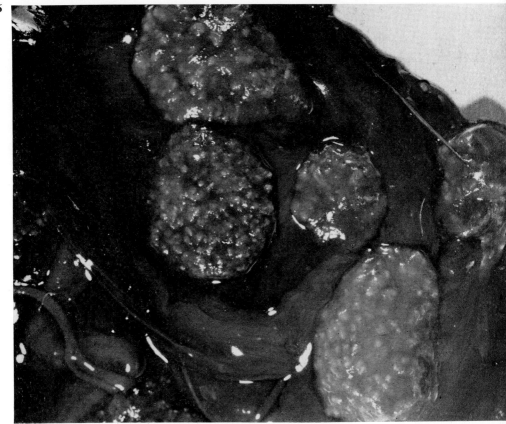

7 Enzootic abortion of ewes (EAE). Note the thickened parchment-like placenta and the well-developed fresh lamb.

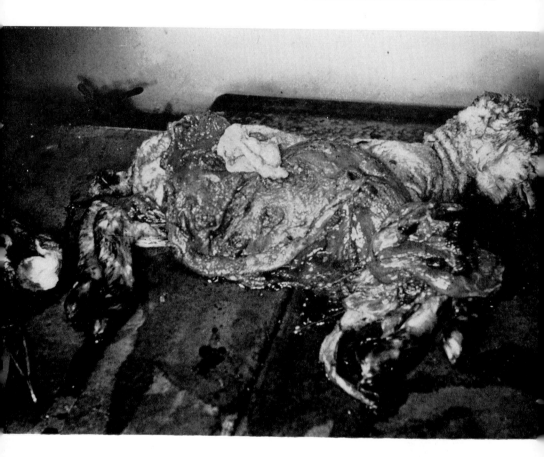

Post-mortem Findings The majority of cases show no gross abnormalities though pneumonia appears to precipitate death. Long standing cases have a degree of enlargement of the brain.

Diagnosis The coarse tremor is fairly characteristic of Border disease. In the absence of 'shakers' a precise diagnosis requires the laboratory examination of several young lambs during the first month or so of life.

Treatment and Prevention Though a transmissible agent has been shown to cause the disease its nature is still unknown and therefore control measures at present must be based on rigorous culling and hygienic flock management.

NASAL CATARRH (Cold)

This condition appears sporadically in hill flocks and is characterised by discharge from the nose and eyes and by coughing. It is obviously infectious and spreads more or less quickly through the flock. Occasional animals may die from pneumonia but in most cases losses are few and the condition generally disappears after a few months.

The cause is unknown but is probably a virus. There is no effective treatment but ewes affected with pneumonia can be treated with antibiotics with advantage. Affected animals should be handled as little as possible and gathering avoided.

PROLAPSE OF THE VAGINA

This condition is seen sporadically in one or two ewes in many lowground flocks as the lambing date approaches. While usually only a few ewes are affected, on occasion the numbers can be serious.

The cause is unknown but it generally occurs in ewes in very good condition. Treatment is palliative. Replacement of the prolapse and an attempt to retain it in position by tying a few strands of wool across the vulva is sometimes successful. An apparatus has been marketed which is claimed to be effective. If the prolapse persists it should be dressed with a bland ointment to prevent drying and ulceration.

PROLAPSE OF THE INTESTINES

On occasion ewes will be found dead with their intestines protruding from the vagina. Again the cause is obscure. The ewe may be seen pressing as if lambing, then the bowel suddenly appears from the vulva. Death is almost immediate. On humane grounds, any animal not dying at once should be killed where she lies. On no account try to get her to a slaughterhouse alive.

CEREBROCORTICAL NECROSIS (CCN)

The name of this disease is only likely to be encountered on a laboratory report or a veterinarian's diagnosis as there is no colloquial name for the condition, which has only been recognised in the last few years. While not usually serious, in that losses are rarely heavy, the disease is by no means uncommon. It is an acute disease affecting the brain and unless treated very early is fatal in one to three days.

SYMPTOMS   Early signs are varied but are usually of nervous origin, with twitching of the ears and face, unsteady gait, staggering and falling. The animal becomes blind and may press its head against a wall or fence, separating itself from the rest of the flock. The condition rapidly worsens and the animal falls on its side and is quite unable to rise though it continues to show signs of consciousness of its surroundings. Convulsive struggling follows with the head being drawn back over the withers which may actually be touched by the back of the head. If the head is forced into the normal position it rapidly returns to this abnormal posture.

CAUSE   The cause is not known but the response to vitamin B_1 (thiamine) leads to the conclusion that a deficiency of this vitamin is involved. Some experimental evidence supports this assumption. The conditions leading to the development of the disease are not known and while cases are frequently associated with scouring and worm infestation the fact that the disease also occurs in housed calves which are worm-free would appear to indicate that worms are not involved. Younger sheep are usually affected, the condition being rare in anything older than 18 months.

The disease may be readily confused with staggers, sturdy, and louping-ill and many cases are dismissed as one or other of these conditions. Diagnosis is, however, readily established in the laboratory by microscopic examination of the brain, but it is essential that the laboratory get the specimen within a few hours of death because of the rapid decomposition of the brain tissue after death.

TREATMENT   If the disease is recognised in the early stages before the brain damage has gone too far, an injection of thiamine into the vein by a veterinary surgeon will give a reasonable number of cures. In more advanced cases the disease can be arrested and a degree of recovery takes place, though the animal may remain blind or unable to swallow. The treatment does, however, allow the animal to be sufficiently revived to be removed to the slaughterhouse for normal slaughter.

PREVENTION   In the absence of more exact knowledge of the cause no preventive treatment is possible. When more than one case occurs, the condition may be arrested by injecting the other animals open to risk with thiamine.

URINARY CALCULI (Stone; Gravel)

This disease is a well-known hazard of feeding lambs and is also encountered in rams. The cause is the partial or complete blockage of the urinary tract between the bladder and the outside. The trouble is only seen in wedders and rams; females are never affected because of the shorter straight tube from the bladder.

CAUSE While some of the causes of the formation of these stones or calculi are known, it is sometimes difficult to determine their cause. They are almost invariably associated with the feeding of concentrates and it is known that, where the ratio of the phosphorus to calcium in the ration is high, there is great danger of this condition resulting. Unfortunately, many grains and proteins used for feeding have this fault of low calcium and high phosphorus. In other cases oxalates and silica may be involved. Oestrogens fed or implanted as growth accelerators can give rise to soft mucoid stones which can effectively block the urethra.

SYMPTOMS The animal is uneasy and restless, and may stand straining in the attitude of urination. Colicky signs may be seen with the animal kicking at its belly. At such times a greatly reduced trickle of urine may be seen. The animal loses its appetite and becomes noticeably ill. The abdomen is distended. Usually the bladder ruptures and death occurs. But in those cases where enough urine can escape under pressure to prevent rupture, the damming back of the remaining urine results in the destruction of the kidneys.

POST-MORTEM FINDINGS The abdomen is often full of urine from the ruptured bladder which may, however, still be intact but grossly distended and blood-splashed. The lining is usually very inflamed and often gritty. Careful dissection of the outlet will reveal the stoppage. The carcase has a very characteristic smell of urine.

TREATMENT This is rarely of value and on slaughter the carcase is likely to be condemned because of the urine in the circulation. 'Dribblers' do sometimes respond to relaxing drugs and operation is possible. This operation may enable the lamb to be fattened.

PREVENTION Rations must be carefully compounded to give excess calcium over phosphorus. Unlimited fresh cold water must be available at all times and it may be worthwhile adding salt to the ration at the rate of 5 per cent to 10 per cent if cases occur. This is said to reduce the incidence of the condition appreciably. Great care must be taken if oestrogens are used and only the minimum dose administered.

BRIGHT BLINDNESS

This condition has been reported in the last few years though it appears to have been recognised in certain hill areas in northern England for some time. An incidence of 5 per cent has been recorded in some flocks. The disease has been seen in Scotland.

Both eyes are affected, giving the animal a noticeably staring, 'glass-eyed' appearance. There is no smoky skin over the eyeball in this condition but the pupil is markedly dilated. Affected sheep show an abnormally alert appearance. The condition is not curable and appears to be worst on poor moors with heavy bracken growth; there is evidence to suggest that the blindness may be the result of eating bracken.

ACIDOSIS

The term acidosis is given to a rather ill-defined disease characterised by quite sudden death. The contents of the rumen show a strong acid reaction.

CAUSE The condition almost always results from overfeeding or sudden change to a grain feed. Barley is particularly significant.

CONDITIONS OF OCCURRENCE The disease is seen when animals are housed and fed cereals, particularly when a large proportion of barley is included and the change made too suddenly. The condition is also seen when sheep are moved to a barley stubble where there has been a degree of wastage. With young animals 10-14 days may elapse before deaths occur, presumably because it takes this time for the animals to acquire a taste for the grain and to seek it out in preference to grass.

SYMPTOMS Affected sheep are often found dead but may have been ill for a few hours. They are dull and separate themselves from the rest of the flock standing with the head lowered and often with regurgitated fluid dribbling from the mouth. They quickly collapse and die.

POST-MORTEM FINDINGS There are no characteristic changes in the carcase but whole grain is often present in the abomasum and chemical tests will show the rumen contents to be strongly acid in reaction.

PREVENTION Avoid management which can result in sheep overeating grain, particularly barley.

Ecto-Parasites

KED INFESTATION

The sheep ked (*Melophagus ovinus*) is a wingless insect which resembles an enormous louse, measuring up to a quarter inch in length. The parasite passes its whole life on the sheep which is the only animal affected.

LIFE HISTORY The female gives birth to larvae which are enclosed in a membrane. The larva is attached to the wool fibres and emerges in about 21 days as a young immature ked. They reproduce in about 14 days. The insect lives about four and a half months.

The ked is a bloodsucker and heavy infestations can produce considerable irritation, particularly during the winter when they are most numerous. The parasite is very active and can be seen moving quickly through the wool. They transfer quickly to human clothing and invariably make their way upwards. After handling infected sheep the shepherd will often find the parasite under his jacket lapels. Keds are frequently called 'ticks' in areas where ticks do not exist and this can be misleading.

CONTROL Because of their residual activity, modern dips have practically wiped out the ked. Any lethal dip with residual activity of more than 30 days will eliminate the parasite from the flock provided all sheep are dipped and none left to form a focus of infection.

LOUSE INFESTATION

Two types of lice are commonly found on sheep in Scotland:
1 The biting louse (*Damalinea ovis*);
2 The sucking louse (*Linognathus ovillus, Linognathus pedalis*).

Undoubtedly the most important louse in Scotland is *Damalinea ovis*—the body louse. For many years lice have been of minor importance largely thanks to the effectiveness of the chlorinated hydrocarbon dips and the fact that dipping was compulsory. Unfortunately, in recent years this louse has developed resistance to the chlorinated hydrocarbon type of dip and severe outbreaks of infestation occurred, even when dipping had been conscientiously carried out. However, about this time organo-phosphorus dips were introduced and proved effective against this parasite. The ability of certain parasites to develop resistance to drugs used in their control is, however, an ever-present danger.

LIFE HISTORY Lice do not live for longer than a week if removed from the sheep. This is important as obviously if all the lice on all the sheep in the flock are killed the parasite could be eliminated. The eggs or 'nits' are attached to the base of a wool fibre and hatch in 7–12 days. The young lice begin laying 14–20 days after hatching. Thus the cycle from egg to egg may be as short as three weeks. Multiplication is therefore very rapid under suitable conditions. Transmission is by contact, either direct or by 'scratching' posts.

CONDITIONS OF OCCURRENCE   Louse infestation is essentially a disease of the winter months. Parasites, both internal and external, tend to increase in numbers when the host's resistance is lowered from deficiencies, poorer nutrition and adverse weather conditions.

SYMPTOMS   Louse infestation is usually accompanied by obvious signs of skin irritation, the affected animals rubbing and scratching on fence posts, etc. In this way they break and remove the wool and affected animals are readily spotted on a casual inspection of the flock. *Damalinea* is, however, a very small and transparent louse and may be readily overlooked unless a magnifying glass is used. When only a few animals are affected the infestation is sometimes confused with scrapie.

While the infestation is quite common in certain areas in animals on free range, the hoggs being especially susceptible, the condition is often at its worst in housed sheep where the loss of wool and condition can be serious.

TREATMENT AND PREVENTION   While in an emergency spraying will give a temporary respite, permanent control can be obtained only by dipping. Modern dips persist for much longer than the one to two weeks required for the eggs to hatch and the young lice come into contact with lethal concentrations of residual dip on emerging from the egg. It is, however, important that all the animals are dipped and that care is taken that no areas of wool or hair are left untreated. Detached tufts of wool may contain eggs which will hatch for some two to three weeks. Sheep, unless recently dipped, should therefore not be introduced for at least a month to pens which have housed infested animals.

SHEEP SCAB

Sheep scab is a readily communicable infestation of sheep by parasitic acari or mites (*Psoroptes conmunes* var. *ovis*) and is a notifiable disease scheduled by the Ministry of Agriculture. No case of sheep scab is known to have occurred in Britain since February 1952 and there is reason to believe that the disease has now been completely eradicated from this country.

LIFE HISTORY   In a well-defined case all stages of development of the sheep scab mite may be found together and are most numerous around the margins of the scab crusts. The mite reaches its maximum size in the adult female stage, when it is an oval whitish creature about one-fortieth of an inch in length with four pairs of relatively long, brownish legs. With a little practice, the adult female is readily visible to the unaided eye when viewed in a strong light against a dark background.

The females lay their eggs in small clusters on the skin at the edges of the scabs and at the base of the wool fibres. During a period of from five to six weeks they deposit up to 100 eggs in all, at a rate of about five each day, after which they die. Eggs normally hatch in one to three days and a six-legged larva emerges. This feeds and after three to four days it moults to become an eight-legged nymph. The nymphs moult after feeding for three or four days and become mature males and pubescent females in the proportion of about one to three. These mate forthwith and after a further two days the young female moults and proceeds to lay eggs one day later. Successive generations are thus separated by intervals of from about 12 to 14 days.

CONDITIONS OF OCCURRENCE Sheep scab mites are not transmissible to any animal other than the sheep and are unable to remain alive for more than two to three weeks when removed from their host. The disease can be acquired only by transference of the parasites from infested sheep or from posts, hurdles, etc, against which such animals have recently rubbed themselves. In its attempts to alleviate the irritation the affected sheep also rubs itself against others and so facilitates the rapid spread of infestation throughout the flock. Animals in poor condition, in which the skin and fleece are deficient in grease, are more susceptible to the disease and in them it assumes a progressive, spreading form.

Progressive or active scab is usually a disease of seasonal incidence and is most prevalent between October and February. In resistant animals, and particularly during the summer months, a latent infestation may occur in which the reproductive rate is low and the mites remain confined to certain sites such as the folds of the groin, the small depression below the eye (infra-orbital fossa) and inside the ears. They do not produce the progressive, spreading lesions until such time as the animals' resistance is lowered, *eg* during winter.

SYMPTOMS The parasites live on the surface of the skin in those areas of the body that are covered by wool. They pierce the skin with their sharp mouth parts to feed upon the tissue juices and thereby produce an exudative, inflammatory reaction accompanied by scab formation and matting and shedding of the wool. The lesions appear typically on the shoulders, back and flanks, but gradually extend throughout the woolly parts. Intense irritation causes the sheep to gnaw and rub the lesion and so aggravates the damage. In advanced cases the constant torment of itch leads to progressive emaciation and finally to the death of the sheep.

DIAGNOSIS Little difficulty should be experienced in recognising the active form of the disease in an affected flock. The lesions which are moist and greasy in appearance are characteristic and are readily distinguishable from other parasitic skin affections, *eg* from the dry scurf and matted wool associated with severe louse infestation. It must be remembered, however, that scab and louse infestations can occur together and consequently the presence of lice on a sheep does not preclude the possibility of the co-existence of scab.

The diagnosis of active scab by a skilled veterinarian is a relatively simple matter. The existence of latent scab, on the other hand, is often very difficult to determine; its diagnosis is of importance particularly in flocks that have been under treatment for active scab and also in those that have been exposed to possible infection. A definite diagnosis depends upon the identification by a veterinarian of the mites in skin-scrapings.

In all cases in which there are the slightest grounds for suspecting the possible occurrence of sheep scab in a flock the information should be conveyed immediately to a police officer who will transmit it to the appropriate veterinary authority.

CONTROL   The control of sheep scab depends upon the complete elimination of all mites from affected animals. This can be accomplished by dipping in baths containing appropriate chemical agents officially approved by the Ministry of Agriculture.

Sheep mange caused by *Sarcoptes scabiei* var. *ovis*, which is also notifiable under the Sheep Scab Order, is confined to the head and other hairy parts and is rarely seen on the fleeced areas. It is characterised by a much drier lesion accompanied by marked thickening of the skin.

There is now evidence that sarcoptic mange in sheep no longer exists in Britain.

TICK INFESTATION

The pasture-tick (*Ixodes ricinus*) is a widely distributed parasite familiar to stockmen throughout the upland and hill regions of Britain where, on account of its frequent association with sheep, it is usually termed the sheep-tick. (NB—In parts of southern England the ked, *Melophagus ovinus* is erroneously referred to as the sheep-tick.) This tick is, however, not a specific parasite of sheep but will feed readily on a wide range of mammalian hosts including deer, hares, dogs, cattle, etc, and even man himself. Out of a life-cycle lasting three years the tick spends less than three weeks as an active parasite. The remainder of its life is passed in an inactive state among the vegetable litter on the ground, but it is able to survive only when there is a high moisture content in the environment. This fact accounts for its virtual restriction to the uncultivated upland areas where vegetation is rough and conditions are humid.

It is difficult to assess how much damage is done by ticks through irritation and blood-sucking, but there is no question of their profound importance as disease carriers, since they are responsible for the transmission of louping-ill, tick-borne fever and tick pyaemia in sheep.

LIFE HISTORY   Eggs are laid on the ground, in cracks and crevices and in the basal mat of the vegetation. From these a six-legged seed-tick or larva emerges and, after a long interval of rest, becomes active one year after the eggs are laid. It climbs to the tips of the herbage to await the opportunity of transferring itself to a sheep or other mammalian host. This achieved, it selects a suitable site and inserts its mouth parts beneath the skin to gorge on blood. After engorgement, which is completed in three to four days, the size is considerably increased and the larva detaches itself and falls to the ground where the next stage of development takes place.

Twelve months later, when the parasite has reached the nymphal stage, a second host is sought and a blood meal is taken during the period of attachment, about four to six days.

In the third year the adult stage is attained and a third blood meal is taken.

Adult female ticks require about ten days to complete feeding and while they are attached to the host the mating process takes place. Finally, the replete, fertilised female returns to the ground where she lays her eggs. Egg-laying is a continuous process lasting four to five weeks, after which the female dies. About 500 to 2,000 eggs in all are deposited to form one mass.

Unfed ticks are flat, oval creatures. The immature stages (larvae and nymphs) are grey-brown in colour, the females reddish-brown and the males dark brown to black. Engorged immature ticks are black in colour while the females are blue-grey. After repletion all stages except the adult male become considerably distended and assume a roundish or ovoid shape and the sizes of larva, nymph and female respectively, are approximately those of a pin-head, a match-head and a pea.

Ticks tend to attach themselves to those areas of the sheep's body which are bare or covered with hair and only rarely penetrate the fleece, except in the neck region. The immature stages are found most frequently on the muzzle, around the lips, on the ears and on the lower parts of the legs, while the adult females are typically seen in the groins, axillae and at the edge of the fleece around the neck. Their presence on the sheep is a seasonal phenomenon. In some areas (*eg* Scottish Borders) sheep are infested only during the spring months, while in others a second season of tick activity occurs in autumn (*eg* western Highlands, northern England and Wales). It has been recognised that ticks in Britain occur in two series, namely spring-active and autumn-active. Those of one series feed at yearly intervals in spring, while the others feed at yearly intervals in autumn. In those districts where spring infestation only is observed the tick-population consists entirely of the spring-active type, while in the western districts generally the populations are mixed and include both types.

During the season of activity all stages may be observed together on the host animal since a population at any given time consists of the current year stages of three separate overlapping generations.

CONTROL Because of the complicated life-cycle of the ticks and the fact that they are capable of feeding indiscriminately on a wide range of mammalian hosts, their control presents a very different problem from that of species-specific parasites such as keds and lice. Protection of the animal by dipping must aim at preventing re-infestation from the pasture. It is a relatively easy matter to kill those ticks which are attached at the time of dipping but, hitherto, no dip has been produced which will give complete protection against re-infestation for more than three weeks. Complete control of a particular seasonal infestation would therefore imply serial dipping at intervals of less than three weeks, but this is obviously an impracticable measure in hill districts, particularly since one of the infestation seasons coincides with lambing time. The problem of complete control must therefore be regarded as unsolved until there are devised dipping preparations capable of extending the protective period. The fact that ticks infect wild fauna and birds is a further factor in preventing eradication.

Since the degree of moisture is a limiting factor to survival on the pasture, it has frequently been stated that some measure of tick control can be afforded through pasture improvement by drainage, elimination of rough herbage by cattle grazing, heather burning, reseeding, etc. Under most hill conditions, however, it is very questionable whether such measures do indeed achieve much, and in any case they can hardly be advocated on account of the considerable practical difficulties involved. The value of such measures lies in their effects on general pasture improvement rather than in their effects relative to pest control. In this connection, however, there is one important feature which should be recognised, namely, that park lands adjacent to tick-infested hills may, upon occasion, become tick-infested. Ticks can persist particularly in the unploughed headrigs and these may prove a great source of trouble because, by maintaining the tick population, they can be the means of introducing tick-borne infections to susceptible park sheep. Similarly, the introduction of infested sheep to grazings far from the infected hill can result in temporary infestation of fields. Thus tick-borne fever and louping-ill can appear in a rather mysterious fashion in permanent low ground pasture.

CUTANEOUS MYIASIS OF SHEEP (Blow-Fly Strike)

'Strike' constitutes a very important economic problem in sheep husbandry and is caused by the invasion of the flesh of the animal by the maggots of certain flies. In Scotland, *Lucilia sericata* (The 'Green Bottle'), *Lucilia caesar* and *Phormia terraenovae* are all involved in 'fly strike'. Much the most important of these is *Lucilia sericata*, which accounts for by far the greatest number of cases of strike in Britain (about 96 per cent). It resembles in its general form the common bluebottle but is smaller in size, about $\frac{3}{8}$ inch in length, and is readily recognisable by its brilliant metallic green colour.

CONDITIONS OF OCCURRENCE In this country blow-fly strike is most prevalent during the period from late May to September. It occurs particularly among sheep which are kept near woods, on enclosed lands containing scrub trees and bushes, or on pastures on which bracken and rank grass are prevalent, as such vegetation affords shelter to the fly. Warmth and moisture encourage the fly's activity and strike is particularly common in warm, sultry weather when the atmosphere is close and humid, or on days when hot sunshine alternates with rain showers.

In Scotland strike was absent or, at most, of very rare occurrence on many of the high hill pastures until about the year 1900, after which time it became very much more prevalent even at the highest grazing altitudes (2,000 to 3,000 ft).

Much attention has been given to the factors which attract the female fly to deposit her eggs on the fleece (so-called 'fly-blow') and it is recognised that she does so in response to the presence of decomposing organic matter on the body of the sheep. Examples of such organic matter are the accumulation of semi-fluid dung in the region of the breech that commonly results from scour; the presence of foot-rot, in which case not only the diseased feet are attractive but also the sides of the chest which become contaminated with discharge from the foot-sores when the sheep is lying down; the bacterial decomposition of skin secretions and matted wool (so-called 'fleece rot' or 'rain rot'); mycotic dermatitis and the presence of wounds such as those that may be inflicted during clipping, and those that occur on the heads of the rams as the result of their fighting, etc.

These various factors, by the odours they produce, prove strongly attractive to the fly which, on settling, lays her eggs on the wool close to the skin, in clusters of 20 to 100 or more. According to different authorities, the total number of eggs deposited by one fly during her lifetime may range from about 500 to 3,000.

The eggs may fail to hatch if the fleece is dry in the vicinity of the egg clusters. This is one of the reasons why warm and humid climatic conditions are conducive to strike, particularly if the fleece is matted and, therefore, more retentive of moisture.

The wounds which result from the penetration of the maggots which hatch from the eggs are themselves highly attractive to the fly: thus a primary strike can make the affected sheep open to a succession of subsequent (secondary) strikes which may occur in rapid succession so that the wretched animal may actually be eaten alive.

LIFE HISTORY The eggs are about one-sixteenth inch long, elongated, and pale yellow in colour, and after a period varying from eight hours to three days they hatch out little yellowish-white maggots which, although they are legless, are very active creatures. The head-part, which is pointed and dark in colour, is armed with two mouth-hooks; the maggot at first feeds on the skin, which is soon punctured, and by using its mouth-hooks, it quickly penetrates the flesh of the sheep on which it then feeds voraciously—this constitutes the 'strike'. Feeding may be completed in as short a period as two or three days (the common limits are two to seven days but the period may be much longer, depending on the temperature and on the amount and suitability of the food). The maggot grows by a succession of moults and when full-grown measures about half an inch in length. The maggots then emerge from the wound and fall to the ground where they burrow into the soil and pupate.

The barrel-shaped puparium consists of the skin of the last maggot stage; it is at first quite light in colour but soon becomes dark brown. The pupation period commonly extends from about 10 to 21 days, after which the adult fly emerges.

The period for the complete life-cycle varies widely and is dependent upon various factors. Under favourable conditions it can be completed in a fortnight—or even less—and several generations of the fly may develop in a single season. Under less favourable conditions two to four weeks or longer may elapse between the completion of each generation, and under cold or other adverse conditions the period may be considerably lengthened. The flies can live a month or even longer and are capable of long ranges of flight (up to 10 miles), even against a strong wind, if this brings to them an attractive odour. Mature larvae which develop at the end of summer do not pupate immediately but hibernate as larvae and so maintain the life-cycle throughout the winter. They pupate the next year and emerge as the first adult generation of the next warm season.

While the length of the life-cycle of the maggot fly varies widely under different environmental conditions, the periods of its various stages might, approximately, be stated as follows:

Incubation of the egg	8 hours to 3 days
Feeding and growth of the maggot	2 to 7 days
Pupation	10 to 21 days

SYMPTOMS The early signs of strike are readily apparent to the observant shepherd. The sheep is flustered and agitated; when the hind parts (a very common site) are affected there may be forcible stamping of the hind legs and vigorous wagging of the tail, or there may be attempts to gnaw at, or rub, the affected parts; the gait may be uncertain and aimless, or the sheep may stand still with the head drooping in a state of misery and dejection. In many cases there is a tendency to wander away from the flock and to hide in bracken or other deep cover.

On close examination a nauseous stench is evident and there is matting and discolouration of moist patches of wool over, or in close proximity to, the strike wound in which the burrowing maggots will be found. A ragged inflamed wound, the discharge from which is highly alkaline, develops quickly. Bodily strength and condition are rapidly reduced and, in extensive infestation, death may result in a few days.

CURATIVE TREATMENT The two main objects in the treatment of blow-fly strike are (*a*) the removal and destruction of the maggots, (*b*) the promotion of the healing of the wound and (*c*) the prevention of restrike.

For the treatment of fly strike either a proprietary remedy or a fly dip diluted to the recommended strength should be used.

PREVENTIVE TREATMENT It is important to prevent or at least minimise the factors which render the sheep attractive to the blow-fly.

TREATMENT OF WOUNDS, ETC All wounds should be repeatedly dressed with a protective and antiseptic application (*see* above); foot-rot sores also require attention. Every one of the maggots should, if possible, be destroyed at the time curative treatment is applied.

DISPOSAL OF CARCASES It is important to ensure the effective disposal of carrion, and particularly of the maggot-infested carcase of a struck sheep, so that the maggots are prevented from pupating and completing their life-cycle. Simple burial of the carcase may not prevent their burrowing upwards to the surface layers of the soil; affected carcases should, therefore, be covered with quicklime or soaked in a strong solution of a reliable disinfectant before burial which should be as deep as possible.

PREVENTION OF SCOURS While complete immersion in a reliable anti-fly dip is a very valuable preventive measure, dipping is effective only if the sheep are relatively clean; it serves little purpose if scouring has occurred and the fleece has become grossly fouled in the region of the breech. Scouring is commonly due to worm-infestation and periodic worm treatment can thus indirectly prove an important factor in the prevention of strike.

'DAGGING' AND 'CRUTCHING' 'Dirty' sheep should be 'dagged', *ie* the soiled fleece, often matted and loaded with dung, removed by shears. The entire flock including the lambs may be 'crutched'. This important preventive measure consists in closely clipping the wool, not only in the region of the breech but also on the inner sides of the thighs and over the rump immediately above the tail; adult sheep can be 'crutched' with advantage just before the first anti-fly dipping (or spraying), about a month or so before clipping-time, at which time the lambs may also be done.

DIPPING The appropriate times for anti-fly dipping vary with locality and with the prevailing climatic conditions. The first protective dip should, of course, be given shortly before the 'blow-fly season' is expected to begin, but an early spell of warm, muggy weather may be an indication to dip sooner than usual. Certainly it is important that dipping be carried out before the sheep are struck.

In a season where a large number of blow-fly strikes occur before shearing-time, it may be necessary to dip or spray—the lambs especially, since they are more susceptible to blow-fly than the adult sheep. Strikes on ewes should be treated as described. If severe it may be worthwhile bringing forward the date of clipping, but crutching may be done with advantage when the sheep are gathered for the first anti-fly dipping (*see* also Dipping, page 88).

SPRAYING AND JETTING Spraying and jetting may be done instead of dipping at the start of the blow-fly season. Power-driven portable sprays are effective and are economic of labour and chemical. Specially formulated sprays must always be used, as dips are not generally suitable for this form of application.

The control of blow-fly strike is largely dependent upon constant vigilance and general good shepherding during the fly season. The tendency for struck sheep to wander and seclude themselves greatly increases the shepherd's task, but it is essential that the affected sheep is spotted and the condition treated at the earliest possible moment.

NOSE MAGGOT INFESTATION

Losses caused by the sheep nasal fly (*oestrus ovis*) are not regarded as important and the condition rarely occurs in Scotland.

CAUSE The adult fly is about half an inch in length and greyish brown in colour (rather bumblebee-like) and is active during the warm months of the year.

LIFE HISTORY The tiny maggots are dropped into the nostril of the sheep one at a time. They crawl up into the nasal passages, where part of their life is spent, then migrate to the sinuses to complete their development. They then leave the sheep and pupate in the soil. The time taken for this development is given as 1–11 months.

SYMPTOMS When the fly is on the wing in summer sheep show signs of anxiety and hide their nostrils in tufts of grass or each others fleece. In light infestations no other sign develops, but in severe cases nasal catarrh may be seen. Pneumonia is an occasional sequel.

There is no satisfactory method of prevention or treatment.

DIPPING

The process of dipping by total immersion of the sheep in a bath containing an anti-parasitic agent was introduced during the earlier half of the last century and developed rapidly with the spread of sheep farming in the new colonial countries. It soon replaced the old practices of 'smearing' and 'pouring' and until recently, has been the only effective means of controlling the skin parasites of sheep. In recent years, however, attempts have been made to replace dipping by sprays or showers, and supplementary measures such as dusting with powders and smearing with salves have been employed, particularly for the protection of lambs against tick infestation. In this country total immersion is the only effective method for the control of sheep scab.

Insecticides may be classified, according to their mode of action, into:
   (1) Contact poisons
   (2) Stomach poisons
   (3) Respiratory poisons
   (4) Dessicants
   (5) Systemic insecticides

The value of a sheep dip depends to a considerable degree upon (a) the readiness with which the anti-parasitic agent may be distributed through the fleece and (b) the persistence of its effective action ('residual activity') in the fleece.

About 1945 gamma B.H.C. (a chlorinated hydrocarbon) revolutionised dipping because of its very high degree of efficiency and persistence. Because of this the control of sheep scab by a single dipping was made possible. In the early 1950s another chlorinated hydrocarbon, dieldrin, was introduced and during the next 15 years this was widely used for the control of maggot-fly, lice and keds. Unfortunately, dieldrin is absorbed through the skin of the sheep and stored in the fat and concern regarding possible ill effects to the consumer caused its withdrawal. At the time of withdrawal, however, the sheep louse *Damalinea ovis* appeared as a resistant strain, so dieldrin was no longer effective for control of lice. Fortunately, the emergence of the organo-phosphorus dips gave us a new and effective weapon against external parasites.

The introduction of the chlorinated synthetics revolutionised our dipping procedure because, although the older insecticides can be relied upon to destroy the active parasites, they are not sufficiently persistent to kill eggs and pupae when these hatch out. With the older insecticides, *eg* arsenic, etc, the period of activity in the fleece was so short that it had expired before all the young parasites had hatched. It was therefore necessary to give two dippings, the first of which could be relied upon to kill all the active parasites, and the second to kill those parasites which at the time of the first dipping and for some time thereafter were still unhatched. The two dippings had to be spaced so that the interval between them was long enough to cover the period of incubation but short enough to ensure the destruction of the young parasites before they, in turn, became sexually mature and so capable of reproducing a new generation.

The costly and laborious procedure of 'double dipping' has been obviated by the introduction of the synthetics; these have such prolonged periods of residual activity in the fleece that only one dipping is required to ensure the total destruction of infestations of keds, lice or scab-mites.

The method of single dipping in a synthetic has eradicated sheep scab and, if properly applied, could effect the total eradication of both keds and lice from this country. These newer agents have the further important advantage that they avoid the risk attendant upon the use of such substances as arsenic and the carbolics which are poisonous to both man and beast.

Skin parasites of the sheep fall into two classes:

(a) The specific parasites which live their whole life on the sheep and have no free-living phase, *eg* keds, lice and scab-mites. These parasites continuously infest the host-animals throughout the year, but winter is the time when, because of the animals' poorer condition, they multiply very rapidly and produce their most injurious effects. The control of species-specific parasites is relatively easily achieved by the proper dipping of the flock in an organo-phosphorus synthetic wash.

(b) The non-specific parasites, *eg* the ticks and blow-flies, which have a free-living stage and infest the sheep only temporarily. They do not infest the sheep in winter and their attacks are confined to certain recognised periods of the year. The effective control of these parasites is much more difficult because they are not completely dependent upon the sheep; thus, ticks are capable of feeding on a wide range of hosts while blow-flies can develop on carrion. The sheep is therefore at risk to a population of parasites which may be independently maintained, and although dipping affords temporary protection to the sheep, it cannot, in itself, eliminate the parasites.

In Britain dipping times are somewhat loosely grouped into three periods:

(i) *Spring Dipping:* In those districts that are tick-infested it is common practice to dip the ewes about one week before lambing and the hoggs shortly before or shortly after their return to the hill from wintering. This gives a considerable degree of protection against tick-infestation during the earliest weeks of the lambing season, but even with the most effective dipping agents now available the sheep are liable to become re-infested about three weeks later; thus dipping, in itself, can make only a contribution towards the larger problem of effective tick control. Dipping does, however, reduce numbers where ticks are few and gives the animal respite from heavy infestation.

(ii) *Summer Dipping:* This commonly has as its main object protection against blow-fly strike. Dipping should be carried out not less than two weeks and preferably three to four weeks after clipping, by which time the growth of the new wool is sufficient to carry the dipping agent. Summer dipping therefore does not normally start until about the beginning of July and continues into the earlier part of August.

The practice of dipping after clipping is good because the best penetration of the insecticidal agents is then achieved and the active ingredients of the dip-wash last longer. However, in certain seasons blow-fly strike may be troublesome before the sheep are due to be dipped or even before they are clipped. There is evidence that, even with sheep in full fleece, some protection can be afforded by spraying in place of dipping, but further experience is required before the actual worth of spraying with organo-phosphorus insecticides can be closely assessed. Little or no control of lice and keds is achieved by spraying animals in full fleece.

If sheep are scouring, or if their fleeces are heavily contaminated with dung-polluted dip, they are rendered much more susceptible to blow-fly strike. Scours are usually caused by heavy worm-infestation which, however, can be controlled by appropriate measures. The actual dipping process should be kept as clean as possible: the immersion of clean sheep in a dung-polluted dip-wash is worse than useless.

(iii) *Winter Dipping:* Because the old standard-type dips, *eg* arsenic, lime-sulphur, carbolics, etc, afforded only relatively short periods of protection, a further dipping in October or early November has long been practised for the purpose of protecting against the three specific skin-parasites of the sheep, *ie* the scab-mites, keds and lice, during the hard months of the year.

It is highly desirable that this winter dipping should be completed at latest in October so that both ewes and rams may have recovered from the unavoidable disturbance and shock of the whole dipping procedure—*ie* gatherings, forcible immersion, etc—before the breeding season commences. Further, it is best to avoid exposing newly-dipped, soaking-wet sheep (particularly breeding ewes) to the effects of frosty and other inclement weather.

It would appear that in spite of the long residual activity of organo-phosphorus dips, winter dipping is necessary to control lice.

Dips, nowadays, are usually obtained ready-prepared in the form of powder, paste or emulsion and the manufacturer's instructions in respect of the method of mixing and the proper preparation of the bath must be implicitly observed. The preparation of under-strength dips is a penny-wise, pound-foolish policy: on the other hand, increasing the concentration beyond the proper strength is not only wasteful but, when poisonous substances are involved, highly dangerous. The strength of the dip-wash should not be computed by guesswork; the materials must be carefully measured. These are matters of such importance that they must be strongly emphasised.

As a result of dipping and the necessary disturbance which it involves, each year brings its crop of casualties. Some losses are of course unavoidable since there are always some animals which for no obvious reason are unable to withstand the excitement and shock attendant upon the dipping process. On the other hand, many sheep are lost simply through failure to take necessary precautions.

Among the foremost causes of losses are rough treatment and careless handling which produce not only physical injury but also excitement and fear. Inhalation of the wash is more likely to occur in the case of over-excited animals, *eg* those that are thrown head foremost into the wash, or that are introduced in too quick sequence so that one falls on top of another in the bath. Further, cuts and abrasions may prove a source of trouble from bacterial infection since the antiseptic properties of most insecticidal washes are relatively low.

'Dip scald' caused by absorption of the dipping agents by the skin, is a condition for which the particular preparation employed is frequently blamed, but, in fact, it is usually the result of failure to take proper precautions. The factors which increase the degree to which skin absorption occurs include: immediate dipping of hot, recently driven sheep, rapid drying in hot sun, driving immediately after dipping before the sheep have dried, inadequate draining, etc. This last factor is often the result of overcrowding in the draining pens which is undesirable for several reasons. The sheep retain an excess of fluid in the fleece and this drips on to the herbage after their release so that the process is not only wasteful of dip but may lead to poisoning through contamination of pasture; or, when drying is rapid, an excess of the agent is retained in the fleece and this, together with the chafing of the skin resulting from rubbing together of closely packed sheep, can cause scalding.

Losses are also likely to occur (*a*) when sheep are too full when dipped, (*b*) when they are in high condition, (*c*) when they are in very low condition, *eg* heavily infested with roundworms, (*d*) when they are empty and remain undried before nightfall, (*e*) when ewes are dipped at a relatively early stage of pregnancy; as a general rule, dipping can be more safely performed the nearer the ewes are to lambing—provided, of course, that they be carefully handled.

Unfortunately, in spite of the labour and expense involved in dipping a flock of sheep it is all too frequently the case that it does not achieve its purpose of effectively controlling the parasites. This may result from several causes including:

(i) The incorrect mixing of the bath, *ie* failure to obey the printed instructions attached to the preparation, or failure to soften hard water when this is specially advised.

(ii) An insufficient period of immersion. When the animals are hurried through the bath deep penetration of the fleece may not occur and thus the dip is not given a proper chance to come into contact with the parasite.

(iii) The failure to submerge the head obviously affords an opportunity for some parasites to escape destruction and to re-infest the sheep.

(iv) Dipping of excessive numbers of animals without regard to the depletion of the active agent in the wash. Bath exhaustion should be avoided by regular replenishment or, where necessary, complete renewal of the wash.

(v) Foul washes; these are less active as parasiticides and may encourage bacterial infection.

Worm-parasites

Worm Infestation

The parasitic worms infesting sheep may be briefly classified as follows:
    (a) ROUNDWORMS: (nematodes)
    (b) FLAT WORMS: (1) Flukes (Trematodes)
                      (2) Tape Worms (Cestodes)

Of the flat worms, the flukes are very important because two of them cause liver rot and one is also a contributory cause in a serious bacterial infection (*see* Black disease, page 19).

The adult tape worms, except in heavy infestation, seem to cause little disturbance to the health of sheep. The intermediate stage of one of the tape worms of the dog is the cause of 'sturdy' and another causes hydatid disease in man and sheep.

(a) I ROUNDWORMS OF THE ALIMENTARY TRACT

Roundworms belong to various 'orders' and 'families' but as, with a few exceptions which will be dealt with separately, they give rise to much the same symptoms, the scientific classification need not concern us here. They are all comparatively tiny, ranging from less than $\frac{1}{4}$–$\frac{3}{4}$ inch in length. Most are very slender and are therefore difficult to see unless separated from the stomach and intestinal contents. When present in large numbers in the stomach and bowel they give rise to scouring and emaciation in the affected animals—parasitic gastro-enteritis (*see* page 94).

Although actual disease and death are important as sources of loss, greater losses result from symptomless lambs carrying a moderate worm burden, with resultant slow maturing and failure to thrive. Any condition which lowers the resistance of the lamb favours the worm, and the heavy worm burden which then builds up is commonly blamed for illness and death, though it is, in fact, a secondary condition. It is therefore important—particularly when older sheep are affected—to examine the management carefully to determine whether or not other factors such as cobalt deficiency, mineral imbalance, overstocking or simply shortage of food might not be incriminated.

Climatic factors also play an important part in the build-up of infestation which can take place very rapidly in conditions favourable to the development and survival of larvae. The factors favouring the parasite are humid warm conditions with good ground cover. Dry weather and bright sunlight, when combined with short herbage, result in a high wastage of the parasite in its free-living stages. The risk of infestation, therefore, varies from year to year and between different areas of the country, even on different fields on the same farm, according to rainfall and temperature. Climatic conditions indeed appear to be a major factor where worm infestation is concerned.

Given the right conditions, animals of all ages can be affected but sheep over a year old strike a balance with the parasites and clinical signs appear only under conditions of stress, *eg* in hill ewes after a severe winter—the so-called black scour—or with specific infestations such as *Haemonchus contortus* infestation, or damage to the large bowel by species such as *Chabertia ovina*. These specialised infestations are considered separately. Parasitic gastro-enteritis is rarely caused by infestation by a single species and is usually the result of a mixed infestation, though one species may predominate.

LIFE HISTORY These worms do not multiply inside the sheep and each worm must be picked up by the grazing animal as an 'infective stage' larva. While there are divergences in the life histories of the different disease-producing strongyloid worms, it is fortunate for our present purpose that the life-cycles of all these worms (with the outstanding exception of *Nematodirus*) are essentially the same and can therefore be described in general terms.

Each fertilised female worm produces an enormous number of eggs—several thousand may be deposited daily. Thus a heavily-infested sheep may, on a conservative estimate, pass out on to the pasture several million eggs daily for several consecutive months. It has been recorded that adult sheep, maintained apart from all possible re-infestation, continued to expel roundworm eggs at an undiminished rate for a period of 20 months.

The eggs, which are microscopic in size, are deposited by the sheep in its droppings and, within about 24 hours, when temperatures are suitable, they hatch out minute larvae. The larvae on hatching are, at first, delicate creatures susceptible to unfavourable influences such as dryness, hot sunshine, cold, and lack of oxygen. They soon moult, however, and pass into the second larval stage and, in turn, into the third or infective-stage larva which is relatively highly resistant to adverse conditions. The development of the infective-stage larva may in very favourable conditions be completed within a week after the eggs are deposited on the pastures, but may take much longer.

The infective-stage larva, unlike its immature forms (the first and second-stage larvae), is unable to feed and must subsist on the food reserves stored in its body; when these reserves are exhausted the larva dies from starvation. The larva, although capable of considerable movement, is encased in a protective sheath and is resistant to adverse influences. Under suitable climatic conditions it will climb up the leaves of the pasture plants and is thus more readily ingested by the sheep. They are stimulated to ascend the leaves by moderate light and warmth, but are repelled by strong, hot sunshine. Moisture is also necessary for these movements which are, therefore, more active when the light is dull and the atmosphere is warm and humid.

Under unfavourable conditions (*ie* dryness, hot sunshine, darkness, extreme cold) the larvae usually descend to the soil into which they may actually burrow, especially in conditions of drought. Although the infective-stage larvae are susceptible and responsive to these various factors, they are capable of withstanding remarkably low temperatures and can survive even after being frozen solid for several days.

The length of life of an infective larva in the pasture is favoured by (*a*) moisture, (*b*) moderate sunlight, (*c*) moderate temperature and (*d*) the presence of oxygen. Nevertheless these same factors also stimulate the larva's activity and movements and in themselves may soon bring about its rapid exhaustion and death; because the infective larva cannot feed, its energy reserves are strictly limited and can be quickly used up.

On hill grazings where the quality of the pasturage is so poor that only one sheep can be carried on two to five or more acres, it might be supposed that the worm infestation of the flocks is low. But on such sparsely populated pastures the sheep tend to graze over particular areas where they find the most attractive herbage and where they have their wonted 'walks' and lairs. These restricted areas can consequently become heavily contaminated with worm larvae. This fact is of greatest importance for lambs but the potential heavy infestation which can quickly appear in the ewe under conditions of starvation must not be forgotten.

It will be apparent that the persistence of worm infestation in pasture is dependent upon various interacting factors. Under the most favourable conditions only a very small proportion of the infective-stage larvae may continue to live in a pasture for one year or more; the great majority usually perish within about three months and in this country it is probable that most larvae, if they fail to infect their sheep-host, die within one month of their hatching from the egg. However, a proportion will survive for many months.

The infective-stage larva commences its parasitic life as soon as it is ingested by the sheep, when it casts off its sheath and burrows into the wall of the bowel. There it undergoes another moult and after about four days returns to the interior of the gut where, after a final moult, it grows rapidly and becomes sexually mature. Egg-laying does not usually begin until three to four weeks after the ingestion of the larva. The larva may be arrested in the wall of the stomach or bowel as a result of resistance of the sheep. Under stress this resistance may be lowered and the larva will then emerge and become mature.

Parasitic Gastro-Enteritis

CONDITIONS OF OCCURRENCE   Parasitic gastro-enteritis may affect sheep of all ages but it occurs most commonly in lambs from about six weeks of age to one year old. The trouble is usually caused by the combined invasion of worms belonging to several species, and the symptoms in any given outbreak depend to some extent not only upon the severity of the infestation itself but also upon the type of worms which predominate. The worms inhabit the true stomach or the small bowel according to their species.

The disease does not occur early in life when lambs are grazing first year grass, but symptoms can appear when they are on older pasture any time after the lambs are two months old. Up to the age of four to six weeks lambs do not graze a sufficient quantity of herbage to pick up a really heavy infestation, so that scouring in lambs younger than six weeks is not, except in very exceptional cases, caused by worms. After this, however, clinical disease can appear at any time, the risk increasing as the pasture becomes more fouled and the grazing scarcer and poorer in quality.

SYMPTOMS   While some outbreaks, particularly when *Nematodirus* is the cause, may be characterised by a sudden disastrous outbreak of scouring in lambs which up to that time had been doing well, most cases show a more gradual onset. The lambs lose their bloom and cease to thrive, faeces become loose and unformed, while some lambs frankly scour and all usually show dirty hindquarters. If left untreated the lambs will rapidly lose condition and in the more severe cases death will occur within a week of the onset of symptoms. In milder outbreaks deaths may be few but recovery will be slow.

POST-MORTEM FINDINGS   Even in severe worm-infestation it is remarkable that relatively little apparent injury is suffered by the lining mucous membrane of the true stomach and bowel; such injury as is present is often limited to congestion and localised, patchy surface inflammation, although on occasion diffuse ulcerative necrosis may be evident. In many cases death results from severe fluid loss from the diarrhoea (dehydration).

DIAGNOSIS   It is important to determine that other factors, *eg* pine or even the system of management, are not the cause of the condition. The presence of worms in dangerous numbers can usually be determined by counting the worm eggs present in the droppings. This must, of course, be done by submitting faeces samples to your veterinary surgeon or to a laboratory. It is important to submit a representative sample, *eg* twelve or more separate samples, since single samples can give misleading results. However, on occasion most of the worms present may be immature and hence not egg-producing, so a low or negative egg count does not rule out the possibility of worm infestation. Post-mortem examination with an actual worm count by the laboratory does, of course, provide definite confirmatory evidence. While egg counts have a useful part to play in diagnosis their limitations must be recognised.

PREVENTIVE MEASURES   Rational measures for the prevention of worm infestation must be based upon a knowledge of the life history and habits of the parasites. Since infestation results from the ingestion of the infective larvae from the pastures and since it was known that at least some of these larvae could remain alive for a period of as long as one year, it was believed that pasture constituted much the most important reservoir of infestation. In recent years, however, opinion on this question has tended to change and newer knowledge suggests that too much importance can be attached to the longevity of free-living larvae. After all, the number of larvae that remain alive in the pastures for upwards of, say, four months is really small—and thereafter progressively declining—and, since all sheep harbour worms, the presence in the pasture of small numbers of residual larvae is of minor importance, with the exception of *Nematodirus*. However, the presence of even a few larvae can lead to a rapid build-up of numbers if susceptible lambs are put on the field.

The majority of free-living larvae die within a few weeks; the great majority die within six weeks to three months and only a comparatively small number survive on pastures for longer than four months.

Resting periods are therefore of some benefit to the pastures, but such a system is not always practicable and, as an expedient, the grazing may be occupied by animals other than the sheep ('alternate-host grazing'). Bovine animals share a few worm species with sheep, but bovines (especially those over two years old) are very satisfactory for alternate-host grazing. These considerations also explain the value of 'mixed grazing' in which different species of animals are grazed on the same pasture at the same time; in this way each species ingests and destroys the other's worm larvae. The contamination of the pasture can be controlled by strategic dosing of the sheep. When sheep, especially lambs or hoggs, are to be moved to clean or well-rested pasture, they should be dosed before moving. The 'build-up' of infestation can thus be delayed. Similarly, routine dosing will limit the number of eggs deposited on permanent grazings. However, the problem is not straightforward and new knowledge continually leads to revision of ideas on this very intricate subject. The emphasis on intensification makes 'resting' techniques of rather academic importance.

CURATIVE TREATMENT   Modern drugs have reached a very high level of efficiency and are dependable and of low toxicity. Some have a very specialised function against particular species, *eg Nematodirus*, so it is important when selecting a drug to have some idea of the predominant worm species. Others are effective against almost all species but the dose may have to be varied. After dosing clinically-affected lamb or hogg flocks, much better results are obtained if the flock can then be moved to clean or rested pasture and in severe cases, or in the absence of clean pasture, box feeding will result in much more rapid recovery.

PREVENTIVE TREATMENT BY DOSING   Management plays a very important part in reducing the risk of clinical symptoms, but as this varies so much under differing systems of husbandry, the problem must be discussed in the context of the individual farm, its geographical location and even the weather at the time. Modern anthelmintics are highly efficient and when properly used can give satisfactory control of parasites.

It is obvious that the dosing of lambs need not be considered till they are six to eight weeks old and then *Nematodirus* is generally the important parasite. Lambs on first year grass need not be dosed till they are three to four months of age and this dosing is largely a preventive measure as even at this stage they rarely carry a burden heavy enough to be really important, especially if the ewes have been dosed before going on to the clean pasture. A general rule, however, not applied too rigorously, is that March-born lambs on contaminated pasture should be dosed against *Nematodirus* in mid-May and mid-June. Thereafter, dosing is governed by the appearance of symptoms and the management system adopted. Lambs being moved to clean pasture should be dosed just before the change. This is particularly important when hoggs are being concentrated on rape or turnips, if outbreaks of lethal 'black scour' are to be avoided. Ewes rarely require dosing and if they do it is generally as a result of some management or nutritional fault or specific infection, *eg Haemonchus contortus*. This is not to say, however, that selected dosing of the ewes may not be sound husbandry: for example, it is customary on some farms to dose the ewes just prior to lambing. This reduces the 'spring rise' in worm egg output and is claimed to reduce materially the contamination of the pastures and to benefit the ewe.

On hill farms lambs need not be dosed till weaning in most cases, though a dosing at the June gathering may be beneficial. Hoggs should be dosed on going to the wintering or on housing and again on returning from the wintering. Again, hill ewes may respond well to dosing before lambing, and if housed, should be dosed when brought in.

Particular attention should be given to the rams which, during the non-breeding periods, are usually pastured on enclosed parks which become heavily worm-infested. Because rams are specially well-nourished they do not commonly show signs of infestation; nevertheless, they are often quite heavily infested and may break down with parasitic gastro-enteritis during the stress of the breeding season. The rams should be treated as a flock by themselves and the advice in respect of dosing, rotational grazing, etc, also applies to them.

Newly-purchased sheep should be treated for worms before they are introduced to the main flock.

The selection of the drug to be used from the many excellent products available may present some difficulty and in cases of doubt your veterinary surgeon should be consulted. Some thought should also be given to the timing and number of the dosings as the economics of the treatment are also important.

SPECIFIC INFESTATIONS

The following conditions present syndromes sufficiently well defined and specific to merit separate consideration.

Nematodirus Disease (Nematodiriasis)

Nematodirus disease is caused by the worms *Nematodirus battus* and *Nematodirus filicollis*. These parasites differ from the majority of the other parasites in this group in that their eggs, particularly those of *N. battus*, develop very slowly. When they reach the infective stage, after four to six months in the case of *N. battus* but 6–12 weeks in the case of *N. filicollis*, they remain within the protective shell unhatched till the following spring. Though the exact mechanism which determines hatching is not fully understood, it appears to be governed by temperature. *N. filicollis* with its shorter incubation period can be found on the pasture throughout the year, so can cause disease outwith the '*Nematodirus* season'. *N. battus* on the other hand has a much shorter season but is often associated with explosive outbreaks.

SYMPTOMS Two forms of the disease exist. The first, which is not uncommon in the Border area, is characterised by a sudden outbreak of scouring in nearly every lamb in the field. The severe diarrhoea results in a very rapid loss of body fluid and lambs may die in three to four days after the onset of symptoms. This severe dehydration causes the lambs to seek water and they congregate round drinking places. The effects are spectacular—lambs which were healthy and thriving fade in a day or two, with complete loss of condition, sunken and discharging eyes and tucked up bellies.

Losses vary according to the severity of the infestation but may be as high as 50 per cent of the lambs in the field; usually, however, 10–20 per cent die. The remainder continue to scour for three or four weeks and then slowly improve. This type of disease occurs characteristically at the end of May and the beginning of June in south Scotland, but may be later further north.

The second type is more insidious in its onset and usually appears in June and July. The bloom goes off the lambs and they begin to scour. The death-rate is much lower in this form of the disease but the loss of condition is equally serious. It is confined to lambs, but once they reach three to four months of age they are rarely affected and adults are completely resistant. The first form of the disease occurs as a result of a sudden massive hatch of the parasite, while the second form is characterised by a slower build-up in worm numbers.

DIAGNOSIS The condition is confined to fields which were grazed by lambs the previous summer or autumn, and an outbreak of scouring on such pasture in late May or June should be regarded with suspicion. Confirmatory diagnosis may depend on a post-mortem examination with identification of the worms.

TREATMENT Several very effective drugs have been developed which will remove these worms. Usually a single dose is sufficient but, if the lambs must be left on the same pasture, a second dose may be necessary in three to four weeks. When clinical symptoms have developed treatment must be followed by box feeding, preferably with a good quality lamb food, if recovery is not to be unduly delayed.

PREVENTION While ewes harbour a few of these parasites, pasture is mainly infected by lambs which, for a short period, pass very large numbers of eggs in their faeces without necessarily showing symptoms. Wherever possible, lambs should be grazed during the danger period on fields which were free from lambs the previous year. A few years ago this was the only method of prevention, but now, by dosing the lambs in May and June, contamination of the pasture can be reduced to manageable proportions. Lambs on other than first year grass should, therefore, be dosed on these two occasions. On first year grass a dose in July is sufficient.

'July Disease'

In late June and in July lambs will frequently scour persistently and show clinical signs strongly suggestive of nematodiriasis. In many such outbreaks, however, worms will be found to be few in number, though the intestine is often swollen and thickened. The condition is not improved by dosing for worms. The cause of this so-called 'July disease' has not been clearly determined, though it can be controlled by clean pasturage and box feeding. It is, however, important to realise that a heavy worm burden is not always the cause and repeated dosing with varying remedies will do more harm than good. A post-mortem examination will clearly differentiate the condition from nematodiriasis.

Haemonchus Contortus

This particular parasite is local in its distribution in Scotland but occurs on both high and low ground. It is a large worm compared to other members of the group, living and developing in the true stomach where it feeds by sucking blood. This characteristic gives the worm an easily recognisable appearance as the blood-filled gut in the female is spirally twisted round the pale ovary giving the so-called 'barber's pole' appearance. This parasite differs from most others in that it can produce severe anaemia and death in adults on adequate nutrition.

SYMPTOMS The main symptoms are pining, a very noticeable anaemia which results from the blood-sucking, and haemorrhage caused by the bites. Where a heavy infestation has been picked up over a short period of time, lambs may not at first lose condition noticeably but the shepherd's attention will be attracted by the animal becoming very breathless on exertion, or even lying down when driven a short distance. Scour is not a symptom of this type of infestation. The signs can appear in lambs within three weeks of exposure to heavy infection.

DIAGNOSIS Because sheep can develop a specific, strong resistance to this parasite, the usual pattern of lambs being affected while the adult stock remains healthy is not generally followed, and the ewes may show marked clinical signs while the lambs appear unaffected. However, signs of marked anaemia in summer should suggest this parasite, particularly in the absence of scouring. The membranes around the eyeball and the lining of the mouth are pale and colourless. As this worm is a very prolific egg producer, worm egg counts are usually very high. Where exposure has been recent, *eg* within 14–21 days, however, the great majority of the parasites may be immature and not yet producing eggs.

POST-MORTEM FINDINGS The carcase is pale and watery, emaciated in more chronic cases, but often in good condition. If the animal has been killed and is still warm, the worms are readily visible to the naked eye when the true stomach is opened. The lining membrane of the stomach shows numerous pinhead bite marks: there are no other lesions present.

TREATMENT Fortunately, this parasite is very sensitive to most anthelmintics and regular dosing will control the disease on infected farms.

Chabertia Ovina

The habitat of this worm is the large intestine where it feeds by biting the lining membrane. It is much thicker than most worms and can be seen attached to the mucous membrane when the larger bowel is opened. Generally speaking it does not appear to be a parasite of major importance but on occasion can become numerous and disease results. The reasons for this build-up are not known.

SYMPTOMS These are the vague signs associated with 'pine'. The disease is only seen in ewes and generally only a small number of the animals in the flock are affected. Scouring is not a symptom.

DIAGNOSIS This can be made only on a post-mortem examination, though it is possible to determine the presence of the parasite from the eggs in the laboratory.

POST-MORTEM FINDINGS Damage is confined to the large intestine, which is thickened and may show shallow ulcers. The worms feed by sucking a plug of bowel into their large mouths and can be seen attached firmly in this way to the bowel wall when the contents are carefully removed.

TREATMENT These worms are susceptible to full doses of most modern anthelmintics and regular dosing will control the parasite satisfactorily.

(a) II ROUNDWORMS OF THE RESPIRATORY TRACT:

Parasitic or Verminous Pneumonia (Husk: Hoose)
Three species of lung worms occur in sheep in Britain:
 (1) *Dictyocaulus filaria*
 (2) *Muellerius capillaris*
 (3) *Protostrongylus rufescens*

(1) Of these the most important is D. *filaria* which is a white, thread-like worm measuring up to three inches in length.

CONDITIONS OF OCCURRENCE Infestation by this parasite is principally confined to lambs under nine months of age and is most prevalent among lowland flocks on intensive grazing in late summer and autumn. Lung worm infestation is commonly associated with parasitic gastro-enteritis.

LIFE HISTORY The life history resembles that of the roundworm of the alimentary tract but with certain differences. The eggs when laid contain embryos which quickly hatch, either in the bronchi or, more usually, in the bowel after the eggs have been swallowed with the bronchial mucus. The larvae are passed out on to the pastures in the expectorate during coughing or sneezing, but more commonly are voided in the droppings. The infective stage is reached in six or seven days. The infective-stage larvae are fairly resistant to cold and dryness, but even under suitable conditions of temperature and moisture they are unlikely to live in the pastures for longer than about three or four months.

The sheep becomes infected by ingesting the larvae which then quickly penetrate the bowel wall and make their way by the lymph and blood vessels to the lungs. There they reach maturity about six weeks after infection.

SYMPTOMS The symptoms are a severe and repeated harsh coughing accompanied by a nasal discharge of thick, sticky mucus. In severe cases, in association with the development of pneumonia and blocking of the smaller bronchi with exudate, breathing may become seriously disturbed. The lamb rapidly becomes emaciated and anaemic and the condition is often further complicated by diarrhoea caused by worm infestation of the stomach and bowel, a symptom with which verminous bronchitis is so often associated. In severe infestations the mortality rate may be considerable.

POST-MORTEM FINDINGS   The carcase is emaciated and anaemic with catarrhal inflammation of the bronchi which contain thick, sometimes blood-stained, exudate in which the worms are massed. Pneumonia, apparent from dark, consolidated patches of the lung, is usually also present.

DIAGNOSIS   The condition may be suspected when numbers of lambs simultaneously show the characteristic cough, but definite diagnosis depends upon the post-mortem finding of large numbers of the worms in the bronchi or the larvae in the faeces. Clinically, the disease may be difficult to distinguish from some forms of pneumonia.

TREATMENT AND PREVENTION   Well-nourished lambs are relatively insusceptible to lung worm infestation; the maintenance of a good level of nutrition is therefore of great importance. Affected lambs should, if possible, be removed from the infested pastures and should be fed generously after dosing against the parasite. The lambs should also be dosed for intestinal worms—at least one commonly used drug is effective against both bowel and lung worms—and dosing should be repeated in three to four weeks.

The two small lung worms, *Muellerius capillaris* and *Protostongylus rufescens*, very commonly affect adult sheep (*M. capillaris* seldom affects lambs under six months old) which, however, often carry heavy infestations of these parasites without showing any ill-effects other than an occasional spasm of coughing. These worms measure about half an inch to one inch in length and are scattered throughout the lungs where they produce small, circumscribed inflammatory lesions that feel like lead shot when the finger is drawn over the surface of the lung.

LIFE HISTORY   The eggs hatch in the lungs of the sheep and first-stage larvae are passed out in the droppings. The larvae enter a snail or slug in which they develop to the infective stage in about 12–14 days. Sheep become infested by accidentally ingesting the snail or slug when grazing. The subsequent development of the parasite is similar to that of *D. filaria*.

TREATMENT   There is no effective treatment for these two parasites.

(b) I. FLAT WORMS

TREMATODES OR FLUKES

Liver Fluke Infestation (Fascioliasis or Liver Rot)

Liver rot, which causes very serious economic loss in the sheep industry, is an acute or chronic disease of the liver and its biliary passages resulting from the invasion of parasitic worms, 'flukes'. It is characterised by inflammatory changes in the liver and, in its chronic forms, by varying degrees of digestive and nutritional disturbance and consequent weakness and general debility.

CAUSE   In this country the disease is caused principally by the common liver fluke, *Fasciola hepatica*; the lesser liver fluke, *Dicrocoelium dendriticum* occurs in some parts of Scotland but is of relatively minor importance.

The common liver fluke is a flattened leaf-shaped creature. Its colour varies from creamy pink to olive green and when mature it measures about an inch in length.

LIFE HISTORY In order to complete its life-cycle, the common liver fluke requires one particular species of snail as its intermediate host. This is a very small mud snail named *Limnaea truncatula*; its shell is sharply pointed and rarely exceeds ¼ inch in length. It occurs in permanent or semi-permanent wet areas, *eg* at the sides of ditches, but does not usually frequent swift-flowing streams, although colonies of the snails are to be found in the calm backwaters of such streams. It has recently been established that although small, scattered populations of snails are widespread in and about permanent shallow water, the large and concentrated populations invariably occur in wet places that upon occasion become dry for periods of weeks, or even of several months. Acid soils, such as make up large areas of hill grazings, are inimical to the snail which thrives best in water from limestone.

The essential phases in the life-history of the fluke are:

(i) The adult fluke in the bile ducts of the sheep produces very large numbers of eggs which pass into the intestine and thence out of the body in the droppings. If the eggs fall on dry ground they die quickly but in wet areas they can remain alive for five months or more, though the majority die in two to three months. The development of the embryo within the egg is inhibited by low temperatures, so that eggs tend to accumulate on pastures during the winter and hatch out in large numbers when the temperature rises in late spring and early summer.

(ii) Usually within a period ranging from nine days to eight weeks (depending on the temperature) the egg hatches and an active larva called a *miracidium* emerges. This swims about vigorously and within a few hours must enter the body of the snail. Should it fail within 24 hours to encounter its specific snail host, the *miracidium* will die.

(iii) The *miracidia* undergo development within the body of the snail and after a period of about 6–7 weeks they ultimately produce new forms called *cercariae* which emerge from the snail and move about rapidly for some hours before encysting upon the herbage. If the conditions are suitably moist and sheltered from the direct rays of the sun, the encysted *cercariae* may remain alive for a period of about eight months or even longer. Although the *cercariae* are remarkably resistant to low temperatures and can resist even continuous freezing for several weeks, it is unlikely that under natural conditions more than a small proportion can live for longer than eight months.

(iv) The encysted *cercariae* are ingested by the grazing sheep, in which, after migrating through the liver for some five or six weeks, they ultimately settle in the bile ducts, where, after a further period of about six or seven weeks, they develop into egg-laying adult flukes. The process of development of the fluke in the body of the sheep, therefore, takes about 12 weeks.

Each *miracidium* that enters the snail may produce 1,000 or more *cercariae*, every one of which is a potential adult fluke. Flukes are hermaphrodite, (*ie* they each possess male and female genital organs) so that each adult individual produces eggs. Flukes may continue to live in the bile ducts for several years and it has been calculated that a single individual may produce more than a million eggs during its lifetime. It is evident, therefore, that even one moderately infested sheep is the means of distributing enormous numbers of fluke eggs and that the reproductive powers of the parasite are very great.

CONDITIONS OF OCCURRENCE   The snail, *L. truncatula*, hibernates or is relatively inactive throughout the winter months, becoming active again during March and April. The eggs which it then produces become a new generation of snails which, in turn, produces eggs some months later—usually about July—while a third generation will become sexually mature in October. It is, therefore, possible that a single snail may become the grandparent of 160,000 snails, and should a colony of, say, 10,000 snails be destroyed with one exception, the survivor could re-populate the area within three months. Therefore, if the weather is wet and the general conditions favourable during the summer, an enormous snail population can build up.

While the adult flukes in the bile ducts continue to deposit eggs throughout the year, the *miricidia* which hatch out are much more likely to find snails in summer when these are more numerous. If snails are not available the eggs falling on the pasture are harmless. As the number of snails builds up in wet summers enormous numbers of *cercariae* may emerge from them to encyst on the herbage in early autumn. In dry years the snail population is much lower and the numbers of *cercariae* are correspondingly reduced.

The fluke requires about three months for its full development in the liver of the sheep, but the first signs of the acute form of the disease resulting from mass infestations of the liver may be evident within a week or two of the sheep picking up a heavy infestation. As would be expected, this is most likely to occur in late summer and autumn. The more chronic form of the disease is seen in the late autumn and winter months.

Acute Type

SYMPTOMS   The acute form of the disease is not uncommon after wet summers. The mass invasion and migration of immature flukes causes inflammation and destruction of the liver and may be superimposed upon a chronic infestation. The affected sheep show dullness and lassitude; the abdomen may be distended and painful on pressure, particularly in the region of the angle formed by the ribs and breast bone. Death often occurs suddenly without the sheep having been noticeably ill and, as in black disease, they may appear to be sleeping.

POST-MORTEM FINDINGS   The abdominal cavity usually contains blood-stained fluid which may also be present in the heart sac. The liver is enlarged and is deep patchy red. It crumbles easily when pressed between the fingers and contains blood clots under the surface; these may be so extensive that the liver capsule ruptures with consequent haemorrhage. The surface just below the capsule shows the wavy tracks of the fluke and, when the liver is cut, these tracks are found throughout the substance.

DIAGNOSIS   A provisional diagnosis can usually be based on the symptoms and confirmed by the post-mortem findings. The condition can be differentiated from black disease only by laboratory tests. Occasionally cases of the acute type have been mistaken for braxy.

Chronic Type

SYMPTOMS   The symptoms of the chronic type are those of lassitude accompanied by progressive weakness and emaciation. Anaemia is invariably present and the membranes of the eye and gums are markedly pale in colour. Dropsical swellings under the lower jaw and on the lower parts of the abdomen are common (the watery 'poke'). The fleece becomes dry and brittle and is broken in appearance; diarrhoea is often present but is seldom severe. If untreated, death from exhaustion may occur in the course of a few months but some cases may make a partial recovery in the spring. It would appear that such recoveries are brought about by the improvement in the sheep's nutritional level which follows the advent of new grass and not to the removal of the infestation. Cases are most commonly seen early in the year, reaching their height at lambing time.

POST-MORTEM FINDINGS   In mild cases the liver may be normal in appearance but on pressure hard cords can be felt which prove to be the dilated biliary passages, the walls of which are thickened, rigid and often gritty. From these passages yellowish-brown bile containing flukes can be pressed out. These formations can also be seen on the surface of the liver as white cords ('pipe-stem liver'). In old chronic cases the bile ducts stand out as white fibrous tubes replacing much of the liver tissue.

DIAGNOSIS   The diagnosis is made on the symptoms and post-mortem findings and by the presence of the eggs of the fluke in the faeces.

PREVENTION AND CONTROL   There are now means of effectively controlling the disease and even reducing it to economic insignificance. Such means are based on the following considerations:
(*a*) Since the snail is essential to the completion of the life-cycle of the fluke, its numbers must be reduced as far as possible.
(*b*) The fluke is harboured by sheep, cattle, deer and rabbits. Control measures must, therefore, be directed against the disease in cattle as well as in sheep by the administration of medicinal agents, and the rabbit population on infested pastures should be reduced to a low level.

It is now known that the snail, *L. truncatula*, is able to resist conditions of drought for remarkably long periods and experiments have shown that some can live in a state of complete dryness for 12 months. The snail is very easily killed by weak solutions of copper sulphate when it is active but not when it is dormant during periods of drought. One part of finely powdered copper sulphate mixed with four parts of dry sand is applied at the rate of 22·5 kilos per hectare (20 lb copper sulphate to the acre) at a time when the snails are active, *eg* in June, to those areas which are known to be breeding grounds of the snail, *eg* ditches, the trampled muddy areas round drinking places and field gates, wet pockets on hill pastures and other areas where there is stagnant water. The treatment should be repeated after an interval of a month or six weeks (in July or August) in order to kill those snails which have hatched from eggs that were not destroyed at the first treatment. The dressing is useful only when the breeding ground of the snail is confined to relatively small areas when it may then be carried out as a yearly routine; the cost of the treatment, apart from other considerations, precludes its general application over wide areas. The Advisory Services should be consulted in determining the breeding grounds of the snail. Copper sulphate at the rate indicated does not affect vegetation but is destructive to fish. It is advisable to keep sheep off the treated areas until rain has washed the copper sulphate from the herbage. Newer products which are lethal to the snail are now available and will probably replace copper sulphate for this purpose.

Where possible, wet areas should be drained and muddy ditches cleaned out. The mud should not be spread on the pasture but rather left in heaps near the ditch bank. It is not advisable to clear out ditches during the late summer or autumn as, at this time, the mud contains *cercaria*-bearing snails and the treatment could have the effect of spreading the infection.

Because of the longevity of the fluke eggs and the part played by the snail as an intermediate host, the periodic resting of infested pastures is impracticable. However, if the areas of greatest risk can be identified, sheep may be removed from them in late summer and autumn. It may be possible to fence off the green springs during the late summer and autumn and in infested fields, to fence off streams or marginal ditches, leaving one drinking place. The Animal Health Division of the Department of Agriculture and Fisheries for Scotland issue a forecast of the likely incidence of fluke for each area of Britain prepared by the Central Veterinary Laboratory at Weybridge.

TREATMENT There is no treatment of value for the acute type of the disease but the presence of fluke infestation in individual sheep is an indication for mass treatment of the whole flock. For many years carbon tetrachloride has been the most effective treatment but now there are several other effective remedies which are very safe indeed. Carbon tetrachloride can be given orally or by injection but it is only effective against mature fluke and the newer remedies, though some claims are made for their effectiveness against immature fluke, will not kill very small parasites. It is, therefore, necessary to repeat the treatment at intervals, especially when the pastures are known to be fluke-infested. These intervals depend on the prevailing conditions of management, and the severity of the outbreak but it can be generally advised, with certain important exceptions which will be mentioned later, that the first treatment may be given in September and thereafter repeated at intervals of about a month or six weeks till February or March, *ie* four or five treatments in all. Treatment after lambing is advisable in badly affected areas to eliminate residual infection in the ewes and prevent contamination of the pasture.

TOXICITY Carbon tetrachloride is a relatively safe drug when administered to sheep but occasionally it produces serious and even fatal toxic effects. The underlying causes of this are not well understood and cannot be attributed to any particular preparation of the drug. From what is known of the conditions under which such poisoning has occurred it is not advisable to dose breeding ewes during the tupping period, to feed concentrates during the week preceding treatment, to give treatment during cold, stormy weather or to subject the sheep to a fatiguing journey shortly before or shortly after being dosed.

For cattle, which are more susceptible than sheep to these untoward effects, hexachlorethane has been advised as a substitute for carbon tetrachloride.

The newer drugs may be used with safety to within a few weeks of lambing and again after lambing and it would seem that the most economic and safe procedure might be to use the cheap carbon tetrachloride in the autumn and one of the newer drugs nearer lambing time where infestation necessitates monthly dosing.

Carbon tetrachloride is not effective against the small liver fluke, *D. dendriticum*, but this is of little consequence since these parasites are of relatively rare occurrence in this country. There is, however, a drug available which will control this particular parasite.

The improvement of the general nutrition of the sheep is as important in the treatment of fluke as it is in all other forms of worm infestation. In view of the very great importance of fluke infestation, the application of control measures should be carried out in consultation with a veterinarian.

(b) II. FLAT WORMS

Cestodes or Tapeworms

Tapeworm Infestation

Two species of tapeworm infest sheep in this country, namely: *Moniezia expansa* and *Moniezia benedeni*. They occur in the small intestine of lambs of up to about six months of age and are much the longest worms found in sheep (specimens measuring 12–15 ft in length are not uncommon) but, in spite of their large size, they appear to cause remarkably little disturbance to health unless present in large numbers.

LIFE HISTORY In order to complete their life-cycle the tapeworms require an intermediate host, a small mite that lives in the grass. The ripe tapeworm segments, which are packed with eggs, break off from the ends of the worms in the bowel and pass out on to the grass with the droppings. There the segments disintegrate and liberate the eggs, which are ingested by the mites. In the body cavity of the mites the eggs develop into an intermediate stage called a *cysticercoid* and lambs are infested by ingesting infected mites as they graze. The tapeworms grow very rapidly in the lamb's bowel and mature segments appear in the droppings about six weeks after infection. Infestations are commonly found between June and September, but the worms do not, as a rule, live longer than three months in the sheep, usually disappearing spontaneously in the late autumn.

The significance of tapeworms on the health of the lamb is still the subject of conjecture. Because of their large size and rapid growth, however, they may divert to their own use some of the lamb's food material and in heavy infestations lambs may become stunted, pot-bellied and generally debilitated. Upon occasion death of the lamb may occur from simple mechanical obstruction caused by a mass of tapeworms impacting the bowel. It is not easy to assess the importance of tapeworm infestation since it is usually accompanied by infestation by nematodes, especially the nematodirus species.

Tapeworm infestation can be controlled by treatment with a copper sulphate and nicotine mixture and there is a specific tapeworm remedy available. Treatment is rarely necessary, however, since the infestation usually clears up spontaneously, and it is rare to find heavy infestations of tapeworms in lambs that are over six months old.

Coenurosis Cerebralis (Sturdy; Gid; Turning Sickness)

CAUSE 'Sturdy' is caused by a cyst, *Coenurus cerebralis*, which is the intermediate stage in the life-cycle of a tapeworm named *Multiceps multiceps* that occurs in the small intestine of dogs and foxes.

It would appear, from the old writings, that sturdy was a disease of common occurrence in the sheep but its incidence now is relatively low. This is probably because the life history of the causal parasite has become well-known to shepherds and consequently the means by which the disease can be easily prevented have been more carefully observed.

LIFE-CYCLE Ripe tapeworm segments, packed with eggs, are voided with the dog's excreta on pasture land; here the segments disintegrate, liberating the worm eggs which contaminate the pasture plants. Sheep pick up the eggs while grazing and the embryos, which hatch from the eggs, burrow through the bowel wall and reach the bloodstream by which they are carried to various parts of the body. Only those that reach the brain or spinal cord will develop into 'sturdy' cysts. The mature cyst as it occurs in the brain is about two ins in diameter; it has a thin, transparent, membranous wall on which several hundred minute, opaque bodies may be seen. Each of these bodies is a potential head of a future tapeworm and each may develop into a complete tapeworm if ingested by a dog or other suitable host.

SYMPTOMS The symptoms of sturdy rarely become evident until about five or six months after the ingestion of the egg, by which time the cyst has markedly increased in size and has begun to exert pressure on the surrounding brain tissue

In general, the animal is nervous and excitable and the facial expression is strained and unnatural. The gait may be unsteady and blundering and convulsive seizures may occur at intervals. Desire for food is soon lost and there is a tendency to wander away from the rest of the flock. The presence of a cyst in the spinal cord may cause partial or complete paralysis.

Generally speaking, when the cyst occurs in one or other of the halves of the fore-brain—the commonest site—the sheep tends to hold its head to the affected side and walks in a circle towards that side. Blindness in one eye may occur, in which case the cyst is likely to be present in the side of the fore-brain opposite the affected eye. Occasionally when the cyst occurs on the surface of the fore-brain its pressure on the overlying bone will render the bone soft and yielding. Such an area may be detected by pressing the tips of the fingers upon the skull.

TREATMENT AND PREVENTION Treatment with drugs is of no avail and the only means of removing the cyst is by surgical operation. Prevention consists in the regular treatment of the farm dogs to keep them free from tapeworms, the eradication of foxes and the strict avoidance of dogs' obtaining the heads of sheep that die from any cause.

Other Tapeworm Cysts

Though *Coenurosis Cerebralis* is the most spectacular condition produced by the intermediate stage of tapeworms of the dog, there are other diseases which are found in the organs of the sheep.

Hydatid Disease

CAUSE The cyst is the intermediate form of the dog tapeworm *Echinococcus granulosis*.

LIFE CYCLE This is the same as for *Coenurus cerebralis* except that the cyst lodges in the liver or lungs. The adult tapeworm is very small, being less than ¼ inch in length so its presence is often unsuspected.

Though the parasite is not common other than locally in Britain and the disease in sheep is not serious, the importance of the parasite lies in the fact that man can be infected by the cysts and the disease can be very serious in the human. The eggs are picked up from the coat of the dog and from contaminated food and vegetables and children may readily become infected in this way. The cyst is very slow growing and symptoms may not appear until years after the egg has been ingested.

Dogs become infected by eating raw offal containing such cysts, each of which can produce hundreds of tapeworms.

TREATMENT AND PREVENTION Dogs should not be fed raw offal and dead sheep should be buried to prevent dogs and foxes eating the infected tissue. Regular dosing of all dogs on the farm will keep infection minimal.

Bladder Worm

This cyst is found as bladders 1–2 ins in diameter hanging from the surface of the liver and the membranes in the abdominal cavity. They cause little harm to the sheep but if eaten by dogs they give rise to a very large tapeworm. When picked up by the sheep in very large numbers the migrating larvae may cause fatal damage in the liver.

Sheep 'Measles'

This condition is rare in Scotland. The cyst lodges in the muscles of the sheep including the muscle of the heart. The cysts are white bodies about the size of a pea but later, they may dry up and become cheesy or gritty nodules in the flesh.

The adult tapeworm, *Taemia ovis*, affects dogs and foxes and is rather small, being 6–12 ins long.

Control of Tapeworm Cysts

It is obvious that there is a close relationship between all these parasites and the sheep and the dog and the risk to the human must also be considered. It is essential, therefore, that sheepdogs be dosed regularly for tapeworms. This is no longer the rather drastic process it once was, for modern drugs are safe and effective and do not sicken the dog in any way. Your veterinary surgeon will supply a stock of a safe, effective remedy which should be used regularly whether or not tapeworm segments are seen. It is important to remember to dose the pet dogs on the farm as well as the sheep dogs.

Allied to this, it is very important that no offal or heads be given to the dogs uncooked; every care must be taken by burying carcases quickly to prevent foxes and dogs eating dead sheep. While *Echinococcal* cysts are not serious parasites of sheep since they grow very slowly and the measures described will eliminate the danger, the disease in man is, however, highly dangerous.

Coccidiosis

CAUSE The disease is caused by a minute single-celled parasite. These parasites are very common in nature and there are few species which are not attacked by one or more types. Each one is however specific to its own host species, *eg* poultry or cattle coccidia cannot affect sheep. The disease is most important when intensive husbandry is practised. Very heavy infestation is necessary to produce clinical symptoms. In early summer the parasite can be seen on microscopic examination of the faeces of healthy thriving lambs, so its mere presence does not indicate disease. Mature sheep are not affected, though they all excrete coccidia in their droppings, thereby acting as reservoirs of infection. The sheep is host to several different species of the parasite.

LIFE HISTORY The parasite differs markedly from the strongyle worm in that it multiplies in the bowel wall of the sheep. It is swallowed as an infective cyst (infective stage) which liberates a number of small parasites when it reaches the bowel. These invade the cells lining the bowel causing damage and there they multiply, finally passing to the exterior as infective cysts. These are the 'coccidia' seen under the microscope. The time taken for the oocysts to become infective on the pasture is dependant on temperature.

SYMPTOMS These are confined to lambs which may show signs of scour. The disease is rarely seen in lambs over 4-5 months old, but symptoms may appear as early as four to six weeks of age. The symptoms are scouring—the motions being chocolate-coloured, offensive and sometimes blood-tinged—unthriftiness, a dry lustreless coat and a tucked-up appearance. The lambs may lose their appetite and rapidly become weaker and die. The death-rate is rarely heavy but the loss of bodily condition is considerable. Recovery may, however, be rapid, particularly if concentrates are fed.

In America the disease is described as essentially one of 'feedlot' lambs and any sudden change of diet can precipitate an attack. It is the only parasitic disease of importance in housed lambs.

In Scotland, the parasite probably plays a part in the scouring associated with nematodirus infestation and the damage done to the bowel together with worm parasites, probably contribute to the condition known as 'July disease'. By this time, however, the damage has been done and increased nourishment in the form of easily digested concentrates is more effective than medicines.

DIAGNOSIS The appearance of bloodstained diarrhoea in lambs too young to be infected with worms should suggest this infestation. It is important, however, to differentiate this condition from basic slag poisoning which also occurs at 4–5 weeks of age.

Under traditional forms of husbandry, clinical signs are rarely attributable to coccidiosis alone, worms being the major factor. In housed lambs, however, outbreaks do occur and it must be remembered that signs of the disease can be present without there being coccidia in the faeces. This is because of the time lag between infection and the development of oocysts. When oocysts are present in large numbers, therefore, the acute phase of the disease has passed.

POST-MORTEM EXAMINATION The lesions are confined to the intestine which is thickened and 'puffy'. Whitish nodules may be seen in the mucus membrane and, in older-standing cases, little 'stalked' bodies, the size often of a small pea, are studded throughout the bowel.

TREATMENT When the disease is suspected, even in the absence of oocysts in the faeces, the administration of drugs of the sulpha group will be helpful. In many cases the diagnosis is made too late for drugs to be very helpful. An attack should be followed by feeding concentrates to affected lambs and providing clean grazing.

PREVENTION Penned lambs should be kept on dry bedding, there should be no abrupt changes of feed and treatment should begin as soon as the first signs are observed; in this case the drug may be added to the drinking water.

The Sheepdog

HEALTH AND WELFARE

No booklet on health in sheep would be complete without some consideration of the indispensable sheepdog. Not only must this animal be healthy, he must be superbly fit and able to stand up to intensive spells of very hard work for weeks on end. His welfare is therefore of paramount importance to his master, yet he is often denied many creature comforts in the mistaken idea that this will make him 'soft'.

Feeding

Obviously fitness depends largely on proper nutrition and when one considers the energy used by the dog in a hard day's work, the significance of an adequate and balanced diet can be appreciated. The consideration must start with the puppy, for if there is neglect at this stage, faulty development may result in rickets and stunting of growth, and this cannot be remedied later. Fortunately milk, particularly fresh milk from a grazing cow, is rich in the minerals and vitamins needed for strong healthy bone, and the puppy should be encouraged to take small supplementary feeds of milk from an early age. Later a reliable puppy food should be provided as well as the milk. Feeds should be given frequently—say four times a day—but never in excess at any one feed. When vitamins A and D are needed—and this is more often the case than not—puppies should be given a good standard preparation at the dose recommended for babies. Crude cheap preparations should not be used, though some preparations specially formulated for dogs are quite satisfactory. Where milk is difficult to obtain, baby foods, and even a good milk substitute, can be used.

Protein is the essential nutrient which is most often deficient in the diet of the adult dog and it is essential that it be fed in adequate amounts. This is in the region of six to eight oz of meat or its equivalent daily. Milk is, of course, also a good source of protein as is sterilised white fish meal and dried skim milk, and these should be used to balance diets consisting largely of carbohydrates. Reliable brands of hound meal and proprietary dog foods are usually carefully balanced to give an adequate diet, but care is necessary in the selection and one must be sure that they do not need reinforcement with meat or milk. Many tinned dog meats are very satisfactory. Brown bread and oatmeal porridge will supply the bulk and the carbohydrate when a concentrated protein is fed. Do not feed white bread. Carcase meat should not be fed to the dogs without prior cooking for reasons which are made clear later.

Housing

It is important that the dogs be given a warm draught-free kennel preferably with an outside run and a pop-hole to the sleeping quarters. The bed should be raised well above floor level and should provide very ample room when occupied by more than one animal, otherwise bullying may result in fighting or in one of the occupants being forced to sleep on the floor. Where an outside run is provided, a raised platform—*eg* an old table—is much appreciated by the dog.

Some form of insulation of the walls and roof is advised and they should be finished in smooth washable material, free from cracks in which vermin could take refuge. The floor too should be impervious and smooth. A deep straw bed which is frequently renewed is recommended, both for warmth and comfort and to avoid the unsightly 'capped elbows' which result when bedding is scarce.

Disease

Sheepdog puppies like any other should be vaccinated against distemper when they are three months old. A combined vaccine will protect against two other common diseases (leptospirosis and hepatitis) at the same time. As these dogs have little contact with infection their resistance may tend to wane after a year or two and a booster dose may be necessary, particularly if distemper appears in the district. Your own veterinary surgeon will advise you. Shepherds familiar with the need for 'boosters' in the ewe will appreciate the reason for this advice.

Parasites

Puppies are often infected with wireworms which are quite large. These worms can be treated at a very early age with very safe medicines but for complete safety and efficiency you should get your veterinary surgeon's advice. On no account give puppies worm capsules intended for older dogs.

The important internal parasites of the adult dog are members of the tapeworm family and, because of danger to the sheep in their intermediate or cystic stage, regular treatment of the dog is a 'must'. Such treatment on a sheep farm must include the pet dogs as well as the working collie, otherwise the benefits will be lost.

The presence of most of these parasites is betrayed by the white contractile segments in fresh faeces, but one species at least is so tiny that these are not seen. Tapeworms do not infect directly from one dog to another but must pass part of their life between dogs in the flesh of another animal in which they appear as cysts or bladders containing white flecks. These cysts must be eaten with the flesh of the intermediate host for the dog to become infected with tapeworms.

While sheep are the intermediate hosts with which we are most concerned, one of these cysts can infect the liver and lungs of the human, causing very serious disease (Hydatid disease). This is not common in Scotland and it is important to see that conditions remain that way. Some cysts cause little inconvenience to the sheep, *eg* the little bladders seen hanging from the membranes in the abdominal cavity, but others again kill. The best known cyst is the one which causes gid or sturdy by locating itself in the brain. Others form their cysts in the muscle, liver and even in the heart. No part of the sheep then can be regarded as safe to feed raw and for this reason meat must be cooked sufficiently to kill all such parasites. Similarly, carcases must be buried promptly before dogs and foxes gain access, because foxes carry many of the dog tapeworms.

Worming should be carried out twice a year and more frequently if the tell-tale segments are seen in the dog's faeces. The choice of drug should be left to your veterinary surgeon, for he has products available which, unlike some of the older remedies, will kill the tapeworms without inconveniencing the dog at all.

External parasites

Dogs suffer from fleas, lice, mange and ticks and it is important that these be dealt with whenever they appear. Dusting powders and shampoos are available which are specially designed for the dog and a reputable product should be used. Dog fleas and lice should never be allowed to become a problem, though odd rabbit and hedgehog fleas will cause scratching on occasion. These, however, do not breed successfully on the dog so their presence is only temporary. When infestation with dog vermin occurs, remember to change and burn the bedding frequently and scrub out the kennels, as well as treating the dog. Dog ticks can be very difficult to eradicate from old buildings where the parasites can readily find shelter.

Mange no longer has the importance it once had because of the highly effective dressings available. These will kill out the infection in one or two applications and are clean and pleasant to use.

Training and Handling Sheepdogs

CHOOSING A DOG

The selection of a suitable dog for training is of vital importance in view of what will be expected of him in his working life. If an 'everyday' dog, in the 'utility' class, is wanted a pup from any reasonably good working parents will be suitable. But if a dog of the highest quality is required, then one should study the pedigree of the puppy and assess the quality of the parents. The prospective trainer should not place too much reliance on the results of trials, important though they may be, but should rather consider the natural ability of the parents. If there is no opportunity to get to know the work of the parents on their home ground, the trials are next best, for here much of the daily work done by dogs on the hill can be seen. Select a pup by a dog which shows good natural ability and control, together with a mild nature, intelligence and hardiness, in preference to one which has attained higher awards as a result of good handling rather than because of its inherent abilities.

Having selected the puppy with the breeding likely to give the necessary working qualities two other points should be looked for, the first being good health and the second good looks. Be sure that the puppy's parents are free from heritable diseases such as progressive retinal atrophy—an affliction not unknown in the breed today—and that they show all the hardy qualities which go to make up the kind of dog which can run all day if necessary.

As the well-known breeder and handler, the late Alexander Millar, said, 'We are not concerned with the physical conformation, show points and the like. We breed from dogs and bitches that have proved themselves to be good workers, intelligent and apt in the handling of sheep. The fact that they may never take a prize for 'type' doesn't matter in the least. Of course, it stands to reason that we only breed from dogs which are physically sound; they could not stand up to the work if there was anything organically wrong with them. Naturally, every man prefers to have a dog with some pretensions to good looks, but at the same time it is not 'looks' that count. As a matter of fact, however, the best sheepdogs today are pretty true to type. Breeding for brains and specialised instinct and stamina has produced a particular type, and working sheepdogs today conform largely to this type. This type is known the world over as the 'working' or 'Border' collie, and it has ousted the 'Old English Sheep Dog' the 'Hillman' and others which were popular in bygone days'.

INITIAL TRAINING

Having procured a puppy of the desired quality training should commence at once, with the simplest of lessons both for the dog and the handler. The first thing to do is to gain the pup's confidence and get him to come to you. Normally this is not difficult as most puppies like company and enjoy being fussed over and petted. But there is always the shy or aloof one which requires a little more attention. Start by feeding him regularly and getting him accustomed to the sound of your voice. Handle him firmly but gently and avoid startling him by shouting, making loud unexpected noises or handling him roughly. He will soon gain in confidence and maturity. A dog's life is a short one and his playing days as a puppy won't last long. During this time, however, he is constantly learning things which will stand him in good stead for the future.

It is quite a good idea to let the puppy have the run of the house. This helps in building up his confidence since he gets to know people, becomes accustomed to strangers calling and to the sound of cars, etc. He will soon learn to accept these comings and goings as one would expect of one of his breeding.

OBEDIENCE

The puppy learns to answer to his name and almost at the same time he is given his first lesson in obedience. If a dog is to be really good he *must* be obedient. When you have gained his confidence the puppy will come to you; now teach him to sit and then to remain sitting while you move away. This may take some time to accomplish but should be practised daily until he understands exactly what is wanted and goes through the exercise showing that he enjoys doing it. Don't make the lessons too long at any one time, or he will grow tired of them and his reaction to your commands will slow down.

As a shepherd always carries a crook or stick, the puppy should become accustomed to it and learn never to be afraid of it. Use the crook when training him to come to you, by tapping the ground at your feet firmly with it so that he learns that there is nothing to fear from it. Once he comes to your feet, strike the ground on either side of him, touch him firmly with the stick, then stroke him with it, at the same time speaking to him and encouraging him.

As he grows and ventures out into the bigger world in and around the farmyard, his every move should be carefully watched for his reactions to the stock in the yard and farm. He may show, even at the age of two or three months, that he has the irresistible inbred urge to herd, by gathering the hens into a corner and keeping them there. He will obviously think this is great fun but he must not be allowed to overdo it. Be content with the fact that he has proved he has the herding instinct and prepare to mould it to your own design.

Every dog differs in nature and temperament and if the trainer is to get the best results he must study each one individually and decide which method is most suited to the particular animal. Generally, the more sensitive dog is easier to train than the more hard-headed, determined one. The latter too often thinks he knows best and refuses to obey his master's commands with the inevitable result that he gives himself more running than is necessary, is harder on his sheep and tries his master's patience, at times beyond endurance. The sensitive dog responds better to the firm and kindly handling of his trainer, is eager to learn and anxious to please and, once thoroughly schooled, will prove a joy to work with and an invaluable and devoted companion. There is no reason to think that this type is in any way less hardy or is less likely to do a full day's work than the hard-headed, determined one. On the other hand if the pup, as he grows, shows a tendency to being a soft, sulky type, too often ready to put his tail between his legs and run for shelter when there is nothing to fear, don't waste your time with him. Breeding produces some curious and inexplicable results, and sometimes puppies with completely different temperaments can come from the same litter. This is why each dog must be studied and treated individually.

INTRODUCTION TO SHEEP

Provided the puppy thrives and learns his first lessons in obedience, he should be introduced to sheep at three to five months old. Again his first reactions should be carefully watched. Don't be surprised, or disappointed, if a little fear or uncertainty shows. If this should happen give him a word of encouragement, bring him up to you, pat him and reassure him. Remember he has confidence in you. It may even be advisable to slip a lead round his neck till he becomes accustomed to the sight and smell of sheep. If you decide that he cannot cope as yet, wait until he is more mature. He will be growing stronger and learning all the time. If, on the other hand, your puppy immediately 'freezes' into the well-known crouching posture of the true sheep dog when he sees sheep, you may feel pleased that the puppy you have chosen has the right instincts strongly developed.

Do not, in any circumstances, allow him to run on sheep until he is strong enough and fast enough to outpace them and still have energy to spare. If he is allowed to run too soon and is unable to head his sheep, he is almost certain to be so frustrated that he will either cut in and allow some of the flock to escape, or give up in disgust. This will retard his progress for he may lose confidence in himself and perhaps in his master also. Though he may be willing to run, you should restrain him until you feel he is able to complete the job he undertakes. Incidentally, you will probably find that before training a puppy you will first of all have to train yourself to be the master of any situation which may arise. Only thus will you command the respect of the dog, and without that respect you will not get very far. Never let him down or offend him and you will find that his respect for you will make him want to please you.

In training him you are helping him to think for himself and thereby to improve his natural instinct to herd sheep. You are not trying to produce a robot which will only work to your commands. The robot type would be of little use on a wide hill where dogs often have to work out of sight of their masters. In fact, it may be said that the robot is of little use anywhere, even in trials when a dog is usually working directly under his master's eye.

Too often we see dogs being stopped as they bring their sheep, when they should be encouraged to come on continuously at an even pace, keeping the sheep on the move without hurrying or upsetting them. The dog which is stopped has to start again and this disrupts the even flow of the run and unsettles the sheep.

So don't give too many commands. Let them be definite and firm without being harsh, and insist that they are obeyed. Insistence on obedience does not mean that you resort to corporal punishment when things go wrong. Understanding and kindness will accomplish much more than the use of the stick. Only when a serious offence is committed should corporal punishment be used, and it should be administered at once when the dog knows the reason for his punishment. There is nothing a dog likes better than a kind word from his master. If he has done badly, the with-holding of that word is punishment in itself, and an even more severe punishment can be administered by completely ignoring the dog for a day or two. Never make the punishment too severe. If you, yourself, are always firm and steady, you will find your dog is too, for the most part, and punishment will seldom be necessary.

TRAINING WITH SHEEP

When you are satisfied that your puppy has grown and developed sufficiently to run on sheep, and that he is willing to go without any forcing or coaxing, put some sheep which are accustomed to a dog into a convenient area and let the puppy away. At this stage an experienced dog should be on hand but a young dog should never be run along with an older one. There are several reasons for this. Usually the older dog resents the intrusion of a young one and will either do his work in a manner which shows his resentment, or he may turn on the young one. The young dog, if put with another, tends to play with it instead of paying attention to the job in hand. Once he has enough confidence in himself to approach and control sheep, however, he will soon prefer work to play. When you are satisfied with his progress and with your ability to stop him at once, whenever necessary, you should start letting him further out and increasing the scope of the tasks and training.

The necessity for insisting on obedience or 'command', as it is generally known among dog handlers, has already been mentioned. Command not only means that a dog must stop immediately, but that he must answer *every* command at once. A dog which will stop instantly but refuses to start again, is just as badly out of command as the one which refuses to stop.

Always give the same command, by the same means (voice or whistle) each time the same move is required. When your young dog starts running on sheep you will soon know by his response, or lack of it, whether your training to date has been successful. If he answers well, encourage him: if he makes mistakes, don't get excited and start shouting or whistling loudly as this will only upset and confuse him. If the situation tends to get out of hand, stop him, call him up and slip on the lead as you speak to him in your normal voice. Use the older dog to get the sheep into order again. You must then decide whether to continue the lesson or to leave it till another day. This should depend on the state of your dog and on what effect the previous attempt has had on him. If you are confident he will stop when required, but is uncertain about what he is required to do when certain commands are given, go closer to the sheep with him. Ask him to come, for example, to your left side, coax him up on that side by repeating the command and move with him.

Well-bred dogs are wonderfully intelligent and apt pupils, and it is sometimes surprising how quickly they learn what their master intends to convey by his different commands and how quickly they respond. In fact, it sometimes seems to the trainer that they are able to read his mind. When this happens it shows that the initial training has been effective, that the intelligent dog has understood, and that his intuitive powers have matured quickly.

If you have difficulty in getting an immediate response to the 'stop' command, try the dog on a long, light but strong cord, attached to his collar with the other end held in the hand. Send him away, and before he has gone the full length of the cord give the 'stop' command. If he does not respond, give the command again, at the same time tightening the cord firmly. He'll stop! A quiet, firm word of reproof may be given before the cord is slackened and he is told to go on, but don't over-scold or frighten him—just remind him who is master. Failure to stop is generally due to over-keenness to work and not to any deliberate attempt to disobey. If the lesson with the long cord is not immediately successful, repeat it until it is.

GATHERING

The dog's instinct is to bring the sheep to his master and a dog with this inherent instinct needs little training in this aspect of his work. He may require to be taught to come at a steady, easy pace without hurrying or harrassing his charges. In sending him to collect his sheep be sure that he keeps off as he approaches and rounds them. His outrun should be like one side of a pear with the sheep at the bottom end. If he tends to come in too sharply, stop him, and keep him off; or better still, keep him off without stopping him. His approach to his sheep *must* be at a steady pace. A dog which can gather and move his sheep steadily and firmly will seldom have much difficulty in controlling them as he brings them to his master, but the dog in too big a hurry will, more often than not, have considerable difficulty and will probably finish with the sheep scattered in all directions.

DRIVING

It is not usually difficult to train a dog to 'gather' his sheep, for the trainer is moulding the dog's natural instinct and ability to his own requirements. It can be much more difficult to get a dog which has the 'gathering' instinct strongly developed to reverse the process and drive sheep away. Do not start training your dog to drive until you are confident you have him in command, and are sure he will stop and flank on either side. Don't be surprised if he is confused at first, for up till now he has been gathering and you are asking him to change direction entirely. The importance of firm confident command cannot be overstated, for without it you will fail in your training. Stop him as he brings the sheep round you, but don't let him lie too long. Keep him moving after his sheep and when he tries to head them, as he surely will, check him and bring him back by your flanking command to the position directly behind his sheep. Keep him walking on and, as long as he is moving reasonably well and driving, continue thus. Don't stop him unless you have to. As in the 'fetch' keep him moving steadily all the time so that the sheep remain docile and more easily controlled. Get him to understand that he is to work at an even steady pace and once he learns this, there should be little difficulty in your control of him and his control of the sheep, except, of course, when sheep are not used to a dog and are wild and difficult. Even in such circumstances, always try to keep yourself and your dog calm and work as quietly and steadily as possible.

SHEDDING

The next step is to teach your dog to 'shed', that is to separate sheep one from another. In hill work it often happens that certain sheep require attention which can only be given in the pens. There is no need to drive all the sheep in the heft, or bunch to the pens, so those not required are shed off and left on their grazings undisturbed. Young dogs with the gathering instinct strongly developed are invariably loath to let any sheep away, but here again, the command you have established will prove itself. As the dog moves to head the sheep being let away, you stop him and bring him in between the two lots. A steady, intelligent dog will soon grasp the idea and, in fact, may become rather keen on shedding. Again it may be necessary to give one particular sheep immediate attention on the hill and, to catch her, a good shedding dog, and especially one which will face up to and wear a single sheep, is indispensable. This also saves driving several sheep a distance to pens and the shepherd walking additional miles. Again be careful not to let the dog rush in in too big a hurry, frightening the sheep. Teach him to face his single sheep steadily and without giving ground. This is perhaps more easily said than done, but a properly trained dog, with confidence in his master and knowing that his master has confidence in him and is in proper command, can make this sometimes difficult task appear easy.

CONCLUSION

In all training and handling of a sheepdog the first essential is complete command or obedience. This should be obtained by gaining the confidence and respect of the dog and not by punishment which should be given only in exceptional circumstances. You will never hammer sense into a dog, but you may easily hammer out what sense he has. Every dog is different: temperament should be studied and the training and handling adjusted to suit it. Before attempting to train a dog, the handler himself must have self-control. Only with the exercise of self-control and with confidence in himself can he impose his will firmly and quietly on his pupil.